HELD BACK by NOTHING

To Amanda

Thanks for your support
I hope you enjoy reading
the book.

John

June 5, 2010

Testimonials

In his new book, *Held Back by Nothing*, author, speaker, long-standing school board trustee, and advocate for special needs students, John Hendry presents an intimate glimpse into the challenges and joys of raising a special needs child. With frank openness and disarming sincerity, Hendry's message of hope and optimism for all children with special needs is compelling. He writes not only from the heart, but also from the knowledge, experience and insight that he has developed personally and professionally over many years. Once you start reading *Held Back by Nothing*, you won't be able to put it down; Hendry has a masterful way of telling a story that grips your heart and inspires you to believe. *Held Back by Nothing* is a "must-read" for all educators and parents of special needs children who want to ensure that every child has the opportunity for a happy, fulfilling and "normal" life.

Linda Fabi, Director of Education
Kitchener, Ontario Canada

The words of United States Secretary of State, Hilary Clinton, "It takes a village to raise a child," ring true in all cases, but never more than for a child with special needs. Parenting an exceptional child requires an ability to forge forward with hope, even in the face of adversity. Supportive family members and friends provide the comfort and encouragement that is vital to successful parenting. As a parent educator, I see the positive difference parents make when they connect with one another. The empathy provided by other parents who have had similar experiences helps to reduce feelings of parenting in isolation. In addition, creating a network of nurturing, supportive family and friends gives your child more opportunities for positive relationships. The value of surrounding yourself and your child with caring people is immeasurable. *Held Back by Nothing* demonstrates countless examples of this principle.

Susan Garber M.A., Parent Education Coordinator
Children's Health Council
Palo Alto, California United States

Held Back by Nothing tells the story of one family's journey of self-discovery as their special needs child reaches outside traditional Special Education beliefs to achieve success in ways that others could only imagine. This journey confirms the belief that all children can excel with the love and support of their family. Every child can succeed and *Held Back by Nothing* proves that.

Jim Berry, Assistant Superintendent
Special Education
Kitchener, Ontario Canada

Held Back by Nothing clearly points out it takes a cooperative effort by parents, teachers, medical practitioners, therapists, and friends to provide the nurturing support the child with challenges needs to be successful. In Australian schools there is considerable funding from government bodies and various organizations to assist schools to help disabled children achieve their potential. There is a strong view that equity for all students is very important, and toward this aim there are numerous programs you can tap into.

Many schools employ a specialist who is trained in delivering programs and services to children with challenges. It is their responsibility to apply to receive the various grants and other funding that is available specifically to achieve this goal. That being said, there is only a finite amount of money available and in most cases is insufficient to meet the needs of all children. Funding for the educational needs of a disabled child in Australia is usually provided by various government programs as well as Independent Disability Support Services depending on the assistance requirements of the child. This process is usually coordinated by the principal or teacher at the school. But above all, the most important thing is treating the student with compassion, love, and respect, recognizing the child, not their disability. The teacher needs to work in unison with the student, the parents, and the agencies involved insuring the student has the greatest opportunity for success. Australia is closely aligned with Canada in regards to this philosophy. However, there is much more to be done.

Coenraad Schoo, Teacher
Mount Gambier, South Australia

HELD BACK by NOTHING

Overcoming the Challenges of Cerebral Palsy

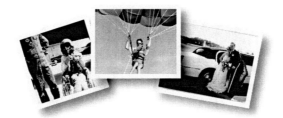

When UNIQUELY NORMAL Becomes EXCEPTIONAL

by JOHN HENDRY

Foreword by Dr. James Israel M.D. F.R.C.S(c)

ENGLEWOOD, CO USA • WWW.ROBERTSROSSPUBLISHING.COM

Held Back by Nothing
How to Overcome the Challenges of Cerebral Palsy and Other Disabilities
When Uniquely Normal Becomes Exceptional
©John Hendry 2010
All Rights Reserved

No portion of this book may be reproduced mechanically, electronically, or by any other means, including photocopying, without written permission of the publisher. It is illegal to copy this book, post it to a website, or distribute it by any other means without permission from the publisher.

Limits of Liability and Disclaimer of Warranty
The author and publisher shall not be liable for your misuse of this material. This book is strictly for informational and educational purposes.

Warning—Disclaimer
The purpose of this book is to educate and entertain. The author and/or publisher do not guarantee that anyone following these techniques, suggestions, tips, ideas, or strategies will become successful. The author and/or publisher shall have neither liability nor responsibility to anyone with respect to any loss or damage caused, or alleged to be caused, directly or indirectly by the information contained in this book.

ISBN: 978-0-9822015-7-2 (paperback)

Library of Congress Control Number: 2010928257

First Edition
Printed in the United States and Canada

Book Design: Design Corps (www.designcorps.us)

Publisher: Roberts & Ross Publishing
Colorado & Florida
www.RobertsRossPublishing.com
(303) 762-1469

Dedication

To Steven and Tanya
For What They Have Accomplished
and
All They Are About To Achieve

Acknowledgments

No one who achieves success does so without acknowledging the help of others. The wise and confident acknowledge this help with gratitude.

Alfred North Whitehead

Writing a book, like any other major project, requires contributions from many individuals. Any attempt to mention all the sources of information would surely result in leaving someone out and require many additional pages. Several individuals that were touched by Steven and shared their memories have my eternal gratitude. They include Steven's Aunt Joan Hackl, Vivian Tambeau, Stephen Swatridge, George Hunsberger, Jeff Poolton, Yumi Hirakawa, Nick Renda, Graham Shantz, Don Poth, Paul Tambeau, and Brandy Duchesne-Martin. A special thanks to a few of our exchange-student daughters who became "sisters" to Steven during their stay in Canada: Gokce Yedidal (nee Gursoy), Turkey; Nikki Wholman (nee Krowitz), Megan Brooke, South Africa; Nastashia Schoo, Australia; and Sandrine Schneider (nee Larrayoz), France. A very special thanks to Yurika Ogata (nee Sawai), Japan. Without the help of these friends and colleagues, this book would not have been possible.

I will be forever grateful to my other two sons, David and Scott, for playing an invaluable role in the progress and development of Steven throughout these years. They made him believe he was equal in every sense of the word.

What can be said to adequately honor the influence and strength of my wife, Linda? She was the stabilizing factor in Steven's life as he journeyed from childhood to a successful young man. Her selfless, unconditional love and her tenacious nurturing planted the seeds of confidence and belief in Steven, and her contribution in the completion of this book was substantial.

A special thank you goes to my writing coach and editor, Kathryn Exner. Her expertise, friendly advice, and patience were invaluable. I could not have completed this monumental undertaking without her guidance.

The publishing of this book wouldn't have been possible without the support of James and Linda Petrozi, as well as the guidance and hard work of Dr. Patricia Ross, Publisher and Senior Editor at Roberts Ross Publishing, and my publicist Jay Heinlein, Heinlein Publishing Services.

Finally, I would be remiss if I didn't acknowledge the significant contribution of Rotary International. Its support of KidsAbility Centre for Child Development (formerly Rotary Children's Centre) laid the foundation on which Steven has built his life. The outstanding staff of caring professionals instilled hope and planted the seeds of success and confidence in him. It was their teachers and therapists who made Steven believe he is uniquely normal.

Contents

	Acknowledgements	ix
	Foreword	1
	Introduction	3
1	And So The Journey Begins	7
2	The First Major Detour	12
3	The Worst of Times and the Best of Times	30
4	Drama, Basketball, and Falling Down Stairs	52
5	Handling Life's Highs and Lows	69
6	Closing in on the Destination	88
7	The End of One Journey—The Beginning of the Next	105
8	They Defied the Odds—So Anything is Possible	118
	About the Author	125
	Appendix: Positive Words to Guide You	127
	Resources, Addresses, and Contacts	131
	Terms of Disability	141

List of Pictures in Chapter Headings:

Chapter 1
Steven at the age of seven weeks

Chapter 2
Steven at seven months—looking very much like every other seven month old baby
Steven's publicity photo as Timmy for the local Easter Seals Fund-Raising Campaign
Steven with his Rotarian, Cecil Omand, attending one of the Christmas parties

Chapter 3
Steven in happier times in his "regular" school
At least two of his surgical procedures required six weeks in a body cast
Steven trying on a fighter pilot's helmet at the London air show

Chapter 4
Steven's high school photo

Chapter 5
Steven with Chicken Pox: Not the way to enjoy Florida

Chapter 6
Steven (in white) and his teammates at a SWAD (Spinners Wheelchair Activity Days) basketball practice. Photograph provided by Pamela Johnston

Chapter 7
Steven enjoying his parasailing adventure
Steven and the love of his life, his wife Tanya
A very happy Steven dancing with his mother

Foreword

Held Back by Nothing is more than just the story of one young man's journey from infancy to adulthood. It is a story of courage, determination, and the unstoppable positive attitude of an individual who refused to let his disability control his life.

This book highlights the dramatic results that can be achieved when the family, friends, and medical community collaborate to provide a child with cohesive support. Held Back by Nothing confirms my belief in the supreme importance of such a supportive environment in the life of any child with physical or intellectual challenges.

It is absolutely essential for these children to have a positive framework around them, particularly when they must undergo treatment. Each member of the support team plays a key role in delivering the same message to the child so there is no confusion. In addition, the child feels more confident when they receive similar messages.

The author also makes a very critical point when he states that while it is important to have a support team and collaborative dialogue, final decisions regarding the child must be made by the parents (or the child if they are of legal age). It is prudent to listen to all the advice given and consider it carefully, but only the parents know the true limitations of the child.

Steven Hendry was a patient of mine for several years and he epitomizes what is possible when a child with a disability is surrounded by a collaborative support team. His approach to surgery was unlike most children I dealt with at the time. While he would probably have preferred not having any surgical procedure, he accepted the situation and made the best of it. Prior to surgery he asked so many questions I often felt like he was the consultant. After the procedure he would follow the advice given regardless of the discomfort and often painful recovery period. His consistently positive attitude was astounding.

How did he develop such a positive attitude? How was he always able to muster a smile in the face of his impending surgery? I am convinced beyond any doubt that the reason Steven is able to approach life's situations with confidence is because of the positive environment in which he was brought up, and the support of so many others both at home and at school, as well as his medical doctors and therapists.

Held Back by Nothing is filled with heartwarming examples of situations every family of a child with disabilities can relate to and draw important guidance from. The section on resources is packed full with useful Web sites and contact information for your reference. If you are able to use just one idea from this book, it could dramatically improve the chances of a successful future for your child.

Dr. James Israel, M.D.
Chief of Medical Staff/Vice President Medical Affairs (retired)
Orthopedic Surgeon (retired)
Grand River Hospital, Kitchener, Ontario, Canada

Introduction

Don't let go of your dreams. If you have determination and belief in your dreams, you will succeed in spite of your desire to let go.

Catherine Pulsifer

It seems like only yesterday that Steven made his entrance into the world. From the very beginning he proved he was a fighter, meeting every challenge with tenacity and determination. Born premature, his body so frail he wasn't expected to survive the night, but he defied the odds and won his first battle. Diagnosed with the condition cerebral palsy at the age of two, the experts painted a bleak future for him including the possibility of his being confined to a wheelchair for the rest of his life—again he beat the odds.

Determined to walk on his own, he pushed his body to the limit in order to gain the strength and agility to be able to walk with the aid of crutches. Armed with an unstoppable positive attitude, reinforced by a supportive family, friends, and medical community, Steven once again demonstrated his mettle by walking away from his wheelchair.

School posed another set of challenges for him. In his first year the reports indicated he would not be able to read or write like other children thereby seriously impacting his future and ability to be independent. Fortunately he was too young to understand or read the reports, so he approached his future in the same manner as any other youngster. School wasn't easy for him, but like his peers he worked hard and found success in his studies. He learned to adapt.

Steven never allowed anyone to set limits on his life. He could never be described as a spectator; he is definitely a participant. He meets every challenge head-on with confidence and the unshakable belief that he can do anything if he puts his mind to it. He also is well aware of his ability and limitations. And he acknowledges the importance of having the support of those close to him, inspiring him to reach beyond his ability.

Throughout his life he has faced discrimination and bias against individuals with disabilities. Integrity has been a big part of his life. He has never used his disability as a means to an end; he has always entered a challenging situation through the front door, even if it means losing an opportunity. To his credit he has spent the past several years trying to improve the world of accessibility for others facing challenges in their lives. Today both Steven and his wife Tanya volunteer hundreds of hours each year with a variety of groups at KidsAbility in Waterloo, Ontario.

With Steven's birth, I became a parent who had to learn how to deal with the day-to-day challenges of raising a child with special needs. As Steven grew older, troubling situations such as major surgical procedures, discrimination, patronizing comments and actions, and potential problems that arose at school, had to be faced and dealt with. Then in 1983 I was elected to the role of public school trustee with a subsequent membership on a special-education advisory committee. Both are positions I have held for many years. In the capacities of parent and trustee, I came to know many children with a wide range of special needs and exceptionalities, many more challenging than our son's. What I came to realize and appreciate was the untapped potential and abilities of children even though they dealt with a daunting spectrum of challenges. I saw many normal children trapped in bodies that inhibited their ability to function like their peers.

Over time I noticed how prevalent it was for many people to stereotype children and adults with disabilities, placing assumed limitations on their abilities and stifling their potential. These challenged individuals were frequently discouraged from setting their goals too high and dreaming of a successful life. Those setting the limitations were well-meaning people who were only trying to help; they believed their advice would spare the child and their parent's major disappointment in the future.

INTRODUCTION

Fortunately, I also witnessed individuals who recognized a child's potential and looked beyond the disability, encouraging the child to shoot for the moon, and to be the best he or she could be. In our own situation, with Steven, I saw firsthand a boy who took on every challenge with a positive attitude and steadfast determination. He never allowed the opinions and attitudes of others, whether it was a doctor, therapist, teacher, friend, or family member predetermine how far he could go, or what goals were realistic.

How did he get that way? What made him different than many of his peers with the same condition? The answers to those questions became the basis for this book. I believed that if I could define what had influenced his life, what had insulated him against following a path determined by others, I could help other children as well as their parents. However, first I had to talk to a wide range of parents to gauge their expectations, as well as their fears, when it came to their child's future. I also decided to contact professionals to see how, or if, their attitudes regarding preparing children with disabilities for the future had changed over the past few years.

I found over and over that there are many supports, such as respite programs for parents, that provide a break from the rigors of looking after a child with physical or intellectual challenges. There are also special accommodations at the child's school including scribes for children with physical disabilities and readers for the visually impaired. Resources such as extensive government programs and special education consultants, who devise and plan individualized teaching strategies, are readily available to optimize the child's learning experience. A variety of clinics, children's hospitals, and pre-school therapy programs are available to take care of virtually all the physical needs of the child with a disability. In addition, most school boards provide special-education teachers and teaching assistants throughout elementary school to ensure children with challenges have the same chances for success as every other child. But as these exceptional youngsters progress beyond elementary school, the supports and resources they have come to depend on rapidly begin to diminish, virtually disappearing by the time they reach adulthood. And as I spoke to hundreds of parents of children with disabilities, it became abundantly clear that what troubled them the most was the uncertainty. What kind of future would their sons and daughters face when they become young adults? More than anything else, that overwhelming fear encouraged the need for this book.

Today, more than thirty years after his birth, Steven continues to "make it" with an infectiously assured attitude and unstoppable determination. Despite his difficult start in life, he has gone on to graduate from college, find his life partner, purchase a home, secure a meaningful job, and earn a seat on the board of directors of KidsAbility in Waterloo, Ontario. He has been one of the most positive influences in my life.

The lessons he taught me I now want to share with you. He showed me that every child has potential. Every child can be successful and stretch beyond the limitations others have placed on them. We can help them by fostering attitudes of confidence, determination, and a positive attitude, and most importantly, help them to develop the belief that they can succeed if they reach just a little beyond the place they now occupy in their lives. It's also critical that all the individuals that are a part of their lives believe in them and push them to be the best they can be.

Children deserve the right to a happy, positive, and independent future, whether they are challenged or "normal." They each deserve the right to set lofty goals and follow their dreams. They deserve the right to set their own limitations. My advice to parents of children with challenges is to never settle for anything less than they have the potential to achieve, and never allow anyone to stifle their chances or discourage them from stretching and being the best that they can be. My hope is that you will be as inspired by Steven's story as I have been, and you will find a way to help nurture and raise your child so that they, too, will enter adulthood a positive, confident individual.

CHAPTER ONE

And So the Journey Begins

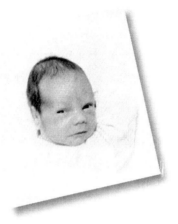

The road of life twists and turns and no two directions are the same. Yet our lessons come from the journey, not the destination.

Don Williams, Jr.

It was in the fall of 1971 that my wife, Linda, and I talked about having a third child. After all, that had been our plan since we were high school sweethearts. The decision wasn't as easy as one would think; Linda had suffered a miscarriage some time after the birth of our two sons, David and Scott, giving cause for second thoughts about having another baby. However, after careful consideration of the risk, we decided to go ahead and complete our family.

The following January, the family doctor confirmed that Linda was expecting, with the due date falling toward the end of September. We had plenty of time to plan and prepare for our new arrival. David and Scott, ages four and seven at the time, were progressing nicely and even though they didn't fully comprehend the pending arrival of a new brother or sister, they were nonetheless excited.

The most popular question of the day, of course, was "Do you want a boy or a girl?" Our response was always the same—we had no preference as long as the baby was healthy. As the time flew by, we wondered if we would have everything in place in for the new arrival. Would we have enough room in our small house? Most people didn't realize Linda was expecting as she wasn't showing any of the obvious signs of pregnancy. We were thrilled she was progressing without any unusual complications. Our excitement grew day by day.

Then, suddenly early one hot July morning our lives changed in a heartbeat. During the night Linda began to feel uncomfortable, experiencing pain in her back. She was sure it wasn't anything serious, perhaps just a routine change in the body, or maybe a touch of the flu. By seven in the morning, however, the discomfort became more pronounced. Not knowing exactly what to do, and probably a little panic-stricken, I decided to seek the help of our close friend and neighbor, Sam (Sandra) Goetz. Sam lived next door making her the first choice in an emergency situation. She was always very calm and confident when it came to handling emergencies; she also had gone through three births of her own.

By the time Sam arrived at the door Linda's water had broken and Sam suggested we get her to the hospital as soon as possible. I called the doctor to let him know what was happening and to have him meet us there.

We arrived at the hospital in near record time. Years later when Linda was recalling the events of that day she said, "On that day I was more nervous about your driving than about my condition." When we arrived, I stopped at the entrance where hospital staff met us, and Linda was lifted onto a gurney. By this time she was in immense pain. Was this pregnancy going to end in tragedy too? Her symptoms were unlike any she had experienced before, even with the previous miscarriage.

I left Linda in the good hands of doctors and nurses while I parked the car. I was very worried so I took my time walking to the hospital in order to get my emotions in check and to psyche myself up to be strong for Linda. I was sure I would have plenty of time while the medical staff examined Linda and made her comfortable, so I was anticipating spending the next several hours in the waiting room before we found out anything. As I walked off the elevator at the maternity ward, the doctor greeted me. "You have a son," he said.

Without missing a beat I said, "Yes, I know, I actually have two sons."

"No," he replied. "I mean you have a son. Linda had a boy."

Needless to say I wasn't prepared for that moment. We were programmed for a September delivery, so this development was hard for all of us to comprehend.

According to the doctor, the delivery started before Linda even entered the elevator and was completed by the time she reached the delivery room. In all, the delivery lasted a mere twenty minutes.

The euphoria of the early arrival of our new son wasn't destined to last very long. The trauma of the delivery and the fact that he was almost three months premature had serious medical implications. Because he was born so quickly, the umbilical cord, which had positioned itself around his neck, temporarily cut off the oxygen to his brain, causing what is called an "oxygen insult." Also, his weight at birth was only two pounds, fifteen ounces, and his lungs had not fully developed.

When I was able to finally look in on him in the incubator, what I saw left a permanent picture in my memory. It was a sight that would break down even the strongest person. Our baby's body appeared to be no bigger than a child's doll. His hands and feet were impossibly small, his skin so thin it was like porcelain. I don't think I have ever seen anything so tiny in my life. He was so small he could easily have fit in the palm of my hand. And the network of tubes connected to that little boy—. We were overcome with emotion and the enormity of a situation we were clearly not ready for.

As the reality of our baby's circumstances began to take hold, our thoughts started to shift from despair and grief to hope—as long as he was alive and breathing on his own there was hope. However a specialist, possibly wanting to help us keep things in perspective, took us aside to tell us that our baby's condition was grave, and that while he would like to give us some hope, we should prepare for the worst. "He probably won't make it through the night," the doctor said quietly. "If he does, the next forty-eight hours will be critical for him as his lungs are not fully developed, and his chest has not completely formed." He was able to provide us with a glimmer of hope; the baby's little heart appeared to be strong. It was at that moment that Linda and I decided that no matter which way things went, it was important that our new son had a name. The name we chose was Steven James.

Despite the doctor's gloomy assessment of his condition and mortality, Steven, even in his fragile condition, somehow found the strength and determination to fight for his survival. There were several ebbs and tides. When he made progress by gaining a little weight, it would give us cause for celebration only to be followed up by a setback in his breathing as a result of his undeveloped lungs. Looking back on this tremendously stressful time, we remember being so worried about Steven that we had no time to think about ourselves.

While Steven was in the hospital we both spent a lot of time at the nursery or the cafeteria. Linda seemed to be there all the time and I was there whenever I could in the evening. The difficult part to deal with was the fact that despite the time needed to be with Steven, we still had two young boys at home. We took great care in making sure they received attention, and also we wanted them to feel we were a family and we were all in this together. We never wanted David or Scott to feel jealous or left out, or worse, we didn't want them ever to feel they weren't important.

We tried to spend as much quality time as possible with the boys and we made an effort to involve them in the planning for Steven's eventual homecoming. Linda would ask David and Scott what they thought he would need when he came home, and occasionally she would take them shopping for baby supplies and encourage them to make suggestions.

On the weekend when Linda was at the hospital I would have a "boys day out" and take the two of them to the mall where we would spend a few hours looking through stores, particularly those with toys and sports equipment, and then relax with a soda in the food court. Every now and then we would treat them to a movie or just go for a drive. It was very taxing on all of us, and at times each of us would require a little positive reinforcement, but we accepted the situation as it was and simply supported each other as we dealt with it in our own way, moment by moment.

Every day we spent as much time at the hospital as we possibly could, keeping a vigil over Steven as he struggled to breathe. Emotionally, we were on a roller coaster ride—one minute we were so thankful he was still alive, but then anger set in that he had to suffer the way he was. Looking around the nursery we saw so many babies, all of them healthy, all of them going home in a few days—all of them but one. At times we almost felt cheated. As the days passed we met a lot of new parents and saw a lot of babies come and go. While some were experiencing the euphoria of a new birth, we were clinging to the hope that our son would survive. It didn't seem fair.

During the next few weeks Steven continued to improve and overcome setbacks. His organs began to mature and started functioning on their own. He was gaining weight and beginning to function more like his little friends in the nursery. Finally, eight weeks after his untimely arrival, we were able to bring Steven home. I remember Linda and me gingerly carrying him out of the hospital. To the casual observer it must have appeared as if he were made of crystal and that the slightest jostle could break him.

Once home I'm sure we checked in on him every hour to make sure he was okay; we left nothing to chance. Day by day, little by little, he continued to show improvement gaining both weight and strength. After a week of sleepless nights, we finally began to feel a little more secure that Steven was in fact progressing.

And so the journey began.

CHAPTER TWO
The First Major Detour

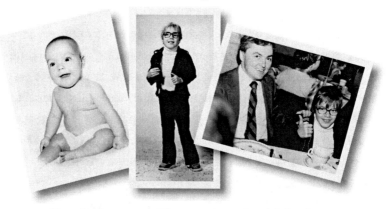

Hope for the moment. There are times when it is hard to believe in the future, when we are temporarily just not brave enough. When this happens, concentrate on the present. Cultivate le petit bonheur (the little happiness) until courage returns. Look forward to the beauty of the next moment, the next hour, the promise of a good meal, sleep, a book, a movie, the likelihood that tonight the stars will shine and tomorrow the sun will shine. Sink roots into the present until the strength grows to think about tomorrow.

Ardis Whitman

By the time he had been home from the hospital for a couple weeks, Steven was progressing like any other baby his age—gaining weight, laughing, smiling, and showing lots of affection. However, we noticed he was having some difficulty sitting up for any length of time, so to give us peace of mind, we decided to call our doctor and have him checked over.

The doctor discovered that Steven had an umbilical hernia that would require surgery to repair. We knew the surgery was necessary but we were nonetheless apprehensive because it seemed like we had just brought him home from the hospital. Steven was still quite tiny and we worried about how he would cope with any surgical procedure at his age, and with his brief history. The doctor told us the procedure was a normal occurrence with some babies and had nothing to do with the complications of his birth. He would be fine. Despite our anxiety, Steven breezed through the procedure and recovered extremely fast. Except for the surgical wound, one would never have known he'd had an operation. Overall, he was a very happy, seemingly normal baby.

LEARNING TO CRAWL

The next few months flew by and his development seemed to be appropriate for a premature infant. He began to recognize a lot of friends and family that seemed to visit on a regular basis. He was a very happy baby and didn't need attention all the time. He always appeared to be quite content just taking everything in around him.

During the next six months, every time Linda took him in the doctor for his regular check-up, she would ask if his development was normal. We noticed he was never at the same stage as other babies his age. The most noticeable characteristic was his inability to crawl. We were told not to be concerned; this was not unusual for a baby born so premature.

Several of our friends had babies in the same time period, so it was quite obvious he was beginning to fall behind the growth and development of their children. But we had faith he was just a little slower and eventually he would catch up. There was no doubt he was a lot easier to care for as we didn't have to chase him around the house or worry about him getting into too much mischief.

Linda wasn't satisfied with the explanation about Steven's lack of progress, so on one of her visits to the pediatrician she asked if there was anything we could do to help him learn to crawl. The suggestion we were given was to assist him with a towel. Yes, a towel! As bizarre as it appeared, it made perfect sense. The idea was to place a towel around his chest and under his arms and hold it above him with just enough strain that it forced him to use his arms and legs without placing too much stress on them. In time it did encourage him to use his limbs a little more and gain strength and confidence.

Eventually he began to pull himself up by himself and after two or three weeks, he started crawling on his hands and knees, never more than a few feet—but it was a start. Unfortunately, it was much easier for him to pull himself around using his arms and hands, literally dragging himself where he wanted to go. We tried to discourage him from that habit, but in the end it was his preferred method of movement from one place to another.

Our decision at the time was to continue working with him every day practicing with the towel, but we were also careful not to frustrate him. We were happy he was motivated enough to want to be mobile. In any event, we believed it was still nothing more than slow development. Eventually he would be crawling around the house, getting into places he wasn't supposed to be, and we would be having fond memories of the "good old days" when he was a lot easier to watch.

Not long after his surgery, I accepted a position with *The Hockey News* in Montreal. That decision forced us to sell our home in Waterloo, leaving our friends and family. The decision wasn't made lightly. As a child, Linda had never even traveled far from her home, so this move was going to be a tremendous change for her. We were going to be leaving everyone we had known all our lives and moving far away to a strange city with a different language. We were starting over, and while Linda wasn't overjoyed, she supported my decision.

I made the move to Montreal first, taking the time to find a place for us to live. Linda was left behind with the mammoth task of packing up our household for transport to Montreal. We couldn't have picked a worse time to move. It was a typical Quebec winter with subzero temperatures and mountains of snow, a grim reminder of just how much I hated this time of year.

It was very lonely living there on my own even if it was just for a couple of weeks. I missed Linda and the boys and spent the nights gazing into space wondering if I had made the right decision. I had no furniture and had to borrow a cot from a neighbor (fortunately for me a neighbor who spoke English). The house had a beautiful fireplace that I used the first night to keep warm. Since there were no curtains on the windows, getting dressed was an adventure. Finally, the wait was over; Linda and the boys arrived and the empty house with no furniture or curtains was soon filled with the warmth and bustle of a family.

By this time, I was in a fairly regular routine at work. As assistant to the publisher, I spent long days at the office in downtown Montreal. *The Hockey News* was published once a week, which meant that several of us had to spend the night before it went to press proofreading copy, selecting the proper photos, and making sure advertisements were in the right place. It was a tedious job, particularly after a long day at the office. The process took several hours, usually lasting late into the night. One evening while preparing the paper, we had an unexpected visitor at the printers. It was René Lévesque, the famous chain-smoking Quebec separatist; he was there to review some of his work for the *Parti Québécois*.

Montreal is a cosmopolitan city with no shortage of beautiful places to visit, so Linda and I spent most of our weekends touring the area with the boys. When we were out and about, Steven was like a magnet. He was friendly with everyone, rendering most admirers defenseless with his engaging smile and constant chatter. He was very comfortable around people and we never discouraged him from talking to strangers as long as we were close by. Settling into our new life in Montreal, we finally started to feel we had made the right decision. Little did we know our lives were about to change forever.

DISCOVERING THE TRUTH

The day started like any other; I got up early in the morning, waited patiently for the commuter train that passed close by our home in suburban Pierrefond, and then endured the crowded half-hour trip into downtown Montreal. But late in the morning, I received a call from Linda who was clearly very upset.

She had decided to take a break from the housework and relax for a few minutes. Linda enjoyed watching documentaries so when her channel surfing happened upon a special feature on young children and babies, she watched intently. The focus of the program was the physical development of a child from infancy to toddler, including the potential effects of premature birth. It included warning signs for a variety of conditions that could cause developmental delays in the child. As Linda recalls it, "A cold shiver ran up my spine and my heart began to pound in my chest. It was as if the program was featuring Steven." The unusually long time it was taking him to walk without support, the difficulty he seemed to have with routine functions such as reaching and holding things, the manner in which he moved even with the support of a table or someone's hand. It all described Steven to a "t."

"Suddenly I had a flashback to our visit to the pediatrician in Kitchener a month earlier," she told me. Our pediatrician was conducting research on premature births and had asked if we would consent to Steven taking part in his study. He had mentioned that Steven's case was very unique given his physical condition at birth and felt the information he would gather from him would possibly help other premature birth children in the future. We were so happy with our miracle and everything the doctors and medical staff at the hospital had done to keep him alive that we consented without hesitation.

Linda immediately called the pediatrician to arrange for an appointment. She took him back to the hospital where he was born. "As I waited with Steven in the examining room," Linda continued, "the doctor left the room to make a call to Montreal on our behalf. He told me he was going to arrange an appointment for Steven with a doctor in Montreal. I thought it was with another pediatrician. During his discussion, I overheard him telling the other doctor he suspected it might be 'CP.' I had no idea what CP stood for. I assumed it was a short form for a medical term. Suddenly, it all made sense; I knew what the doctor was referring to a month earlier. Steven has cerebral palsy!"

Linda is usually the calm one in the family, the one who considers all the facts rationally before reacting. The fact that she was so upset by this realization about Steven signaled that something was definitely wrong. In retrospect, I suppose the coincidence of Linda tuning into that particular program on that day was a good thing as it prepared us for the news we would soon receive from the specialist at Montreal's Children's Hospital.

THE FIRST MAJOR DETOUR

The day we traveled into the city to meet with the doctor and discuss the results of all the tests he had conducted was quite difficult for us. On one hand we wanted and needed definitive answers so that we could make the necessary plans and get on with our lives, but on the other we feared the worst, wondering just how bad the news was going to be. Our worst fears were realized during the consultation as the doctor confirmed Steven's condition was indeed cerebral palsy. The doctor thoroughly explained the condition in layman's terms. The damage had occurred during birth when Steven's brain had been deprived of oxygen for a brief time.

The result in Steven's case was that all four limbs were affected, with one arm and one leg being more affected than the other. The only positive information we received from the doctor was that cerebral palsy was not a progressive condition. However, the normal growth of the child causes ongoing problems that are usually treated through intensive, often painful, therapy or surgery, such as the lengthening of tendons.

> Steven's diagnosis was not confirmed until more than two years after his birth. This situation is consistent with information found on the Ontario Federation for Cerebral Palsy Web site. Diagnosis and confirmation can take anywhere from birth to the age of thee depending on the individual child's brain development. This delay results in valuable treatment time being lost. Meanwhile the child does not develop at the same rate as other children his or her age. The faster you can get an accurate diagnosis, however, the better because the child can start the proper therapy sooner. Parents should not hesitate to have their child examined and tested if they think there is any sort of developmental problem.

We were told that it was too early to tell what the full impact would be on Steven's physical and intellectual development, but unfortunately he would never be able to walk normally. It would take some time, perhaps several years, to determine if he would be restricted to a wheelchair or if he would be able to walk with the assistance of crutches.

As far as Steven's intellectual development was concerned, we would have to wait to see how he advanced as he grew. However, the fact that he was communicating normally at that time was a good sign and other than some "developmental delays," the doctor thought he would probably be okay. Until he attended pre-kindergarten or school, it would be very difficult to determine what other issues he might be facing. Premature children sometimes require a couple of years in school before they catch up to their peers of the same age. When you add cerebral palsy to the equation, the period of delay can be extended considerably in some children.

Immediately following the diagnosis, we began to research cerebral palsy in order to have a clearer understanding of the condition and also to try to rationalize how it could have happened to Steven. We discovered that there are many causes of cerebral palsy, in fact as many as twenty. In Steven's case it was caused by two chance events—his premature birth and a delivery that was too abrupt, causing the oxygen insult to the brain.

Each of us in the family handled the news differently. Since I was working all day and the occasional weekend, it was easier for me to keep occupied and not think about it. David and Scott were still quite young, and perhaps more realistic, accepting the news and moving on. Linda, however, was with Steven all day, so it was always at the forefront of her mind.

I thought what Linda really needed was someone close to her, a friend she could talk to, so I called her best friend, Vivian Tambeau, inviting her to come to Montreal and stay with Linda for a week. She agreed and arrived the following weekend. The time they spent together was therapeutic for Linda and was just what she needed. Having a friend to talk to, to catch up on all the news and gossip from home and to share a few tears with, helped her regroup. "I really went there to try and support Linda through that period, just by being there for her or helping look after the boys so she could have some time to herself to adjust to the fact that this was going to be a life-long condition," Vivian told me later.

In retrospect, the months we lived in Montreal following Steven's diagnosis were the best thing that could have happened for Steven and the rest of the family. We had very few distractions and only a couple neighbors we could call friends, so we spent a lot of quality time together. It gave us the chance to talk about our future and to consider how we would move forward.

OUR BOYS ARE CREATED EQUAL

David and Scott were enrolled in school and were starting to feel comfortable in their new surroundings. They were making friends and putting the disappointment of moving behind them. In time, Linda began to love living in Montreal too. She had made some friends and was beginning to immerse herself in the French culture. This was now her home. Unfortunately, I wasn't as adaptable as the rest of the family. I missed our friends and family back in Ontario and other than my colleagues at *The Hockey News*, I really didn't make any attempt to meet new people in the neighborhood. But as long as Linda was happy and the boys were making progress, I would make an effort to accept the experience.

Wherever we were going to be living, we decided, we were going to raise Steven in the same manner as the other two boys. As difficult as we thought it might be at times, we wanted to make sure Steven was treated as an "equal," and that meant equal in the true sense of the word. He would follow the same rules as his brothers and be disciplined the same. There would be no pity, no feeling sorry for Steven. We were determined to bring him up as a healthy, happy boy. At the same time, we weren't naive; we realized there were obvious limitations and concessions that would have to be considered to accommodate his challenges. I remember trying to explain to David and Scott that while it was nice that they liked to do things for their brother, it was vital that they didn't become too overprotective. It was important for Steven to be exposed to the same difficulties in life as other children his age. We explained to them in whatever why we could that in the long run it would be the best thing for Steven as he matured and faced challenges without his brothers there to help him.

One thing Linda and I insisted on was that we each had the responsibility for watching out for those who would pity Steven in public by giving him money. Unfortunately, we experienced this situation everywhere and all too often, from shopping malls to the park. I always wondered why people wanted to give money to Steven so badly. But their reasons were theirs. It was more important that we stuck to our guns. We told the boys that although it was an act of kindness, it was also ignorance. Our philosophy was that money was earned, not acquired through begging. Unfortunately by giving any child money, even a child with challenges, you are assuming they are either completely helpless or at the very least a case for charity unable to meet basic necessities on their own. Every cent that was given to "that poor little boy" was returned with thanks and appreciation for their kind gesture with the explanation that he is really "quite alright." It was not an easy rule to enforce; telling a little boy he could not have money that was offered to him was definitely not an easy task.

It took some time but the whole family got into a daily routine that worked for each of us. Steven loved to play and get into places he wasn't supposed to be just like every other child. However, unlike every other child, Steven also had to spend time with his mother getting his daily sessions of physical therapy and exercises. The exercises were very uncomfortable for him, and often quite painful, but other than the occasional "ouch," he accepted the stretches and bends without ever complaining. Linda tried to make it a game whenever possible, trying to help him understand all the pain she was causing was in his best interest. Despite his condition, the rigor of the therapy and exercises in no way ever slowed him down. Afterwards, he would forget the pain and carry on like any other two-year-old child.

As if things weren't bad enough that year, we were about to experience yet another abrupt development. *The Hockey News* was about to be sold. The new owners—an established communications firm with a solid management team—were located in New York City. The change in ownership made my position with *The Hockey News* redundant. The news was upsetting at first and not easy for Linda and the boys to accept.

We had sold our home in Waterloo, left our family and friends to start a new life in Montreal, and received the diagnosis of Steven's condition—all in less than eight months. Since I wasn't bilingual, my options were limited. I felt somewhat disillusioned. Had my boss known that the paper was going to be sold when he hired me? Taking a page from my own advice to the boys, I decided to accept the situation and to turn the disappointment into an opportunity.

As with every situation having an impact on our family, Linda and I discussed the options available to us. Our decision was to return to our home in Ontario. I was silently elated; Linda was outwardly disappointed. She was happy to be going back, but at the same time she had embraced Montreal as our new home. We had given up a lot to make the move in the first place, and less than a year later we were going back. David and Scott had mixed feelings. They had finally started to feel like they were fitting in with their friends and at school, but they were excited about moving back home to the place they loved the most. Steven of course couldn't understand what all the fuss was about.

THERAPY'S LONG AND PAINFUL ROAD

As soon as we arrived back in Waterloo, our first priority was getting an appointment with Steven's pediatrician. We were hoping he would allow Steven back into his research project. We trusted the doctor and felt Steven would benefit from the ongoing assessments. The time that had elapsed between our leaving Waterloo and returning was actually short in terms of scheduling appointments with a specialist, so the doctor was happy to fit Steven back into his program.

By now Steven had reached his third birthday and the doctor felt it was time for him to get into the preschool and therapy program at the Rotary Children's Centre in Kitchener. The center focused on providing specialized occupational and physical therapy for a wide variety of exceptionalities including cerebral palsy. When he explained the program and the potential benefits to us, we couldn't wait to enroll Steven. Each day he would attend school in the morning and receive occupational and physical therapy in the afternoon on alternating days. The academic part of the day gave children with disabilities an opportunity to participate in a "head-start" program, allowing them to catch up with other children their age by the time they entered grade one or two.

> Surgery is a common occurrence for children with disabilities, particularly those with cerebral palsy. Cerebral palsy isn't a degenerative condition; the damage that takes place, usually at the time of birth, never gets any worse. However, as the child grows, the muscles and tendons don't always grow at the same rate making surgery necessary to provide a temporary correction. It's only temporary because the child continues to grow, necessitating additional corrective surgery such as the lengthening of tendons or muscle transplants, until the normal growth patterns stop.
>
> The decision to proceed with corrective surgery is usually made in collaboration with the physician, parents, and therapists and when appropriate, the child. Therapists should carefully monitor and document the condition of each child, reporting on a regular basis to a consulting orthopedic surgeon to determine if any changes might be required in the therapy program, or if surgery is necessary in order to help the child.

The therapy sessions were intensive and grueling. Therapists worked on his tendons and muscles in his legs and arms, teaching him to crawl and climb stairs. Eventually they taught him to start walking on his own with the help of a walker. This was a miracle; it was so exciting for us to see him walking. The expression on his face displayed his pride as he slowly and methodically moved along the floor toward us. It brought tears to our eyes. But progress came with a price. The spasticity in his legs and tightness of his tendons resulted in the need to wear special shoes. They looked like normal shoes for the most part, except wires came up from the top, clasping like a bracelet a few inches above his ankles to support his legs and prevent his feet from turning inward.

Three months after his fourth birthday, Steven required surgery to lengthen the tendons in his legs. Cerebral palsy is a condition, not a disease which means in Steven's situation, the damage was done at birth and would not progress. However what does happen is various parts of the body do not grow or mature at the same rate. In Steven's case, the tendons in his legs were most affected. Left unchecked his legs would eventually twist in the hip joint making walking difficult and painful. In time he would not be able to walk at all.

Even though he had to go through several surgical procedures as a child, his positive attitude prevailed. He never protested, and if he had pain he never complained or talked about it. Visiting him in the hospital was at times entertaining as he became a favorite of the nurses. However, it was a bit distressing that he had to be in the hospital so frequently that he and the nurses knew each other by name. His recovery was always quite fast, though, as he seemed to have the ability to heal quickly. During the next several years, Steven endured countless surgical procedures. Our friends would often ask us what it was like for us dealing with Steven's condition day after day. They wondered how we found the emotional strength to cope with the setbacks he would have from time to time. The best response I could give was, "It is like having a different heartache every day."

UNLOCKING THE CHILD WITHIN

The days at the Rotary Children's Centre (now called KidsAbility Centre for Child Development) flew by. Steven looked forward to the arrival of the school bus, driven by his favorite driver, affectionately known to the kids as "Driver Bill." Bill was much more than just the driver of the school bus. He loved kids and felt very comfortable around children with challenges. If a child needed a special kind of equipment or support, Bill would not rest until he was able to help find it. He even found time to occasionally visit with the children at their homes on the weekend.

Driver Bill was an extension of the school and mirrored the attitude that seemed to be displayed by every staff member. They made every effort to engage parents in their child's education and therapy. Staff frequently called parents to give them updates on their child's progress or to make helpful suggestions to follow through with their therapy. They also encouraged parents to visit the school whenever they had an opportunity to do so, giving mothers and fathers the chance to see another side of their child.

The school's academic curriculum was integral. It was designed as a "head-start" program because many children with disabilities are also delayed in their readiness to attend school. With this type of opportunity available, the children were often able to enter the regular school at the same level as their peers.

Linda and I would visit the class from time to time to observe Steven's progress. We found the atmosphere in the class was always upbeat. The teachers were truly gifted when it came to engaging their students in the various activities. If there was one word to describe this classroom, it would be "fluid" as there was always something happening. There was never a dull moment for the teachers and therapists as the children seized every opportunity to enjoy time with each other. The teachers loved their work, engaging the children and making learning fun for them. Giggling and outright laughter seemed to be the norm in the class. It was obvious the children were learning and were happy about it.

OUR OWN LITTLE PIRATE

Shortly after he started attending the center, the teachers and therapists noticed an abnormality in Steven's eyes. He was experiencing a great deal of difficulty tracking. Tracking is the ability to control the fine eye movements required to follow a line of print especially when reading. Children with tracking problems usually lose their place, skip or transpose words, and experience difficulty with comprehension or understanding the subject they are reading. We were told he required surgery to correct the problem, but even with surgery the doctor felt he might have difficulties reading and writing in the future.

Eye problems seemed to become an ongoing part of Steven's life. Soon after, he developed a "squint" caused by one of his eyes turning inward. As a result he had "squint repair" surgery where the doctor performed a procedure to strengthen the eye muscle correcting the condition. During his recovery, he wore an eye patch while the eye healed. We would lovingly tease him, telling him he looked like a little pirate. It was always in fun and had significant importance in the way he felt about himself and how would handle his disability in the future.

Our goal was to help him understand and accept the reality of who he was. He had a disability and that was never going to change; it was a reality—his reality. We told him everyone is different. Not one person in this world is perfect, and there were many individuals who significantly more serious challenges than his. Treating him the same as his older brothers and making sure his brothers also treated him the same as they did each other was critical. He was never to be treated like a victim, and most important, he was never to act like a victim.

Linda and I spent a lot of time helping him understand that people may tease him or stare at him. He had to understand that this would probably happen throughout his life. When Steven asked the obvious question, "Why do people say those things about me?" our reply was that people who say hurtful things or stare usually do not know any better. They are the type of people that would say unkind things to anyone who is different; it had nothing to do with his physical disabilities. The best thing for him to do was ignore it and not draw any further attention by responding. It hurt us to the core that people would be so rude and unkind, but it was more important that Steven develop a strong sense of self and be proud of whom he was.

LEARNING TO FALL

Not only did Steven receive an education at the Rotary Children's Centre School, but Linda and I also benefited. The support we received during that period of Steven's life would go a long way in helping us better comprehend his disability and limitations. It was important for us to fully understand his condition in order to help guide him through the years ahead.

Collectively, the teachers and therapists at the Rotary Centre were amazing with the kids. It was obvious, even to the casual observer, that they loved their jobs and they loved their charges—every student was important and received an equal amount of attention. They each took a personal interest in every child, motivating and encouraging the kids to be the very best that they could be, and most importantly, to believe in themselves. Believing in themselves and establishing strong self-confidence would become essential factors as they journeyed through their lives. It amazed us how the center was able to secure such dedicated and committed teachers and therapists. The nurturing they gave these young pupils would give them the roots to grow and the wings to soar as high as they possibly could.

"It was a really special place with great people," Steven recalls. "It's funny, I don't remember the classroom, but I remember going to physiotherapy sessions in the middle of the day and then heading back to class." It isn't surprising he remembers physiotherapy so vividly; it was very difficult and sometimes painful work. Stretching tendons and working muscles that never seemed to cooperate would not be easy for anyone, yet Steven and his friends who were all of three years old endured it everyday.

Most important, the life skills taught at the center were priceless. I am convinced some of these lessons may have saved Steven's life on numerous occasions over the next few years. Teaching a youngster with cerebral palsy how to fall down without getting hurt is an example of one of these skills. Most people would shake their heads and question the logic in teaching a child to fall down; after all, once you have lost your balance you fall down, right? The truth is, children with cerebral palsy, particularly those who have difficulty walking unassisted, and those who walk with the help of crutches, lose their balance easily and fall down a lot. A bad fall can result in a serious injury, including broken limbs. Since many children with physical disabilities do not have the same sense of timing as others, their reaction time is normally much slower than other children at the same age. As a result, they are not always able to protect themselves in a fall. Teaching them how to safely fall was just one of many skills the children were taught. There are numerous other simple actions we take for granted that are very difficult for a child with a disability to accomplish. Teaching them how to adapt to various situations, even as simple as pulling on their pants or buttoning a shirt or blouse, was very

THE FIRST MAJOR DETOUR

helpful as it allowed them to develop more self-confidence and independence—something they would take with them as they grew older.

Steven loved attending school. Each day he would be up at the crack of dawn, shoveling down his breakfast so he would be ready when Driver Bill arrived to transport him off to school. Sometimes he would stand at the door peering out the window waiting for that familiar Rotary Centre van to pull into the driveway.

When he arrived home from school, we would always talk to him about his day. He loved to talk, so we usually heard every detail, including information we were probably better off without. The subject matter didn't matter in the end, though; it was heartwarming to hear the enthusiasm in his voice. We felt it was important for him to know that we were genuinely interested in what he'd learned, what activities he had participated in, and how his therapy had gone that day. By demonstrating a genuine interest in his experiences at school and encouraging him to keep trying as hard as he possibly could, we would help him develop that sense of pride in himself.

He was always so positive and happy at school that at age three he was chosen to be the "Timmy" for the Easter Seals Campaign. Timmy was the name given to the child who would represent all children with disabilities during the annual fund-raising drive. It was an honor for him although he couldn't quite comprehend the full meaning, and as his parents, we were thrilled and very proud of him.

While he didn't fully understand the honor, that didn't diminish his thorough enjoyment of the experience and benefits. He had an amazing year attending dinners, having his picture in the local paper, and traveling to Canada's Wonderland with a police escort for a day of rides, souvenirs, and the excitement of being treated special by everyone. The Timmy experience planted a seed in Steven—it gave him a fuller comprehension of his uniqueness and abilities—and the confidence it established in him was unbelievable. Even though he already had a positive attitude, the experience definitely reinforced his self-esteem.

It was a big thrill for Steven when he was asked to drop the ceremonial puck at a Kitchener Rangers hockey game before more than four thousand fans. The game marked the end of the Easter Seals campaign, during which thousands of tickets had been sold on a draw for a new car. It was Steven's job to draw the winning ticket. As thrilling as that duty may have been, the real excitement was him being on the ice and shaking hands with the hockey players in front of all the spectators. We were astonished at how poised he was; he showed no signs of any nervousness. A couple of weeks later he was invited to travel to Maple Leaf Gardens in Toronto. He had the chance to meet Hall of Fame hockey legends, Johnny Bower and Lanny McDonald of the Toronto Maple Leafs, and while Steven enjoyed it, I must admit it was more exciting for me. Steven and I also got to have lunch with Canadian actor Don Harron (a.k.a. Charlie Farquharson). Mr. Harron was amazing with Steven and showed a genuine interest in him.

DEVELOPING QUIET CONFIDENCE

At the time, the Rotary Children's Centre was funded for the most part by local Rotary Clubs, with some additional financial support from the government. (Today the Province of Ontario provides most of the funding for what is now KidsAbility Centre with some financial assistance still coming from some Rotary Clubs.) However, Rotary did much more than just donate money; Rotarians also assisted with transportation when families needed to have their children travel out of town for appointments with specialists or to receive treatment unavailable in their hometowns. Rotary participation didn't stop there; they also held annual Christmas parties and spring fishing parties for the children. A Rotarian was assigned to every child on the center's caseload. They would pick the children up from their homes and attend the party with them. It was an incredible experience for both child and Rotarian. In addition, it gave the parents some needed time away from the daily rigors of caring for a child with disabilities.

Steven was very fortunate during his time at the center to have some very caring Rotarians as his "buddies" for the events. One of those buddies was Cecil Omand, now retired Director of Education of the Waterloo Region District School Board. Mr. Omand would pick Steven up at the house, drive him to the fishing party or the annual Christmas party, and spend the entire trip talking about what Steven did at school or what he wanted for Christmas. Although they only saw each other for a few hours a couple times a year, Steven was always made to feel like he was pretty special. The hours he spent with Mr. Omand were memorable to this day.

The result of Steven's Rotary Children's Centre experience was nothing short of miraculous. The teachers and therapists possessed a special gift for inspiring their students. He loved the school, the staff, and the friends he made. When he was told he was about to "graduate" and move into a regular school, he was both disappointed and nervous. Even at his young age, he understood that at the center he was with friends and other children with the same condition and similar developmental issues. In the new school, he would be in a totally foreign environment—a system where nearly all the other students would be "normal"—and it was a little frightening for him. Change is difficult for children; for some it can be a traumatic experience to move from the comfort of familiar surroundings.

During the summer Steven was able to talk to a lot of his neighborhood friends and began to develop a growing sense of adventure and excitement. As September drew near, and the realization that he would be in a "normal" school with "normal" students sank in more fully, his fear gave way to anticipation.

Because we had always treated him exactly like his brothers, he found a quiet confidence in himself. Despite his limitations and exceptionalities, he had developed a strong self-esteem and he was ready to take on this new challenge. Steven always had a remarkable attitude, finding something positive in every setback; for some inexplicable reason, he could see only possibilities. Early on, Steven truly believed he was "uniquely normal." He was the same as every other child: some had pimples, some had allergies, others had learning disabilities—he had cerebral palsy.

He was ready for the next turn in the road.

CHAPTER THREE

The Worst of Times and the Best of Times

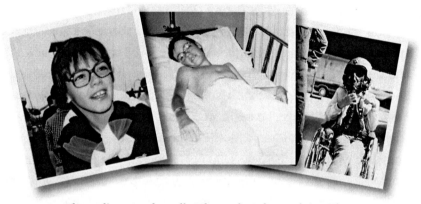

The mediocre teacher tells. The good teacher explains. The superior teacher demonstrates. The great teacher inspires.

William Arthur Ward

Special education programming in the late seventies was evolving, but it still had a long way to go. It had begun to move away from the practice of segregating children with special needs into special classrooms away from the mainstream students even though they all went to the same school. They called it a "congregated class," and the argument for this type of class was that the disabled student would receive the assistance he or she needed in a more controlled environment, away from "normal" students. It was felt this practice would help the child reach his or her potential.

The misguided theory at the time was that children with exceptionalities would benefit from the experience of simply attending a "regular school," even though they weren't really part of it. The broad meaning of "special education" at the time was instruction specifically designed to meet the unique needs of children with various disabilities. The real issue with "special education" was that teachers received some specialized training in teacher's college, but it wasn't enough to deal with the sweeping range of exceptionalities they encountered. In other words, there was no "special ed" distinction in an education degree. So back in the seventies the specialized teachers in charge of instructing boys and girls with challenges were usually very dedicated and to their credit believed all of their students could learn regardless of their disabilities. However, despite these teachers' commitment to their children, they often lacked adequate resources to be effective.

By the late seventies, educational practices had the students with exceptionalities simply integrating back into the classroom, willy-nilly. It was, in a way, the polar opposite of the congregated classroom idea. Students like Steven, or even children with mild to severe learning disabilities, were in the same classroom as everyone else. It didn't matter what kind of exceptionality they had. They were "mainstreamed," and everyone kept their fingers crossed that it would all work out.

It was a rough ride for Steven; I'm not surprised, looking back over the broader history of special education, that in the early years of his primary education, Steven wasn't always able to get the help he needed from his teachers. At first this was a bit of a shock, especially after all the excellent care and instruction he had received at KidsAbility Centre. Children that attended the Centre remained on the case load for the therapists, and education consultants familiar with each child would visit the schools once a month to evaluate their progress and discuss any issues that the teacher might have had either with their academic needs or concerns with their physical situation. Even though the consultant's visit was helpful for the teacher and was of great value to Steven at the time, it didn't provide the support the teacher needed to manage a class with one or more students with challenges.

I recall one parent-teacher meeting we attended when Steven was in grade one. Steven had moved from a congregated class with twelve students into a regular classroom setting at his new school. This was the first opportunity we had to meet with the teacher to discuss his progress and the areas in which he needed help. We attended, expecting an informative discussion with a caring educator, and, quite frankly, we were expecting to hear how hard Steven was trying and how much fun he was to having in the class.

Instead, we found ourselves in a state of constant frustration due to the lack of communication and process when it came to Steven's education. He, like every other child with special needs in the system, had a personal file called an OSR (Ontario Student Record). Pertinent information regarding his progress was documented in this confidential record. Details concerning his learning disability, specific information about the nature and complexity of his physical disabilities, and strategies for effective teaching methods to assist the teacher were part of this very helpful file. Itemized reports from his physiotherapist and occupational therapist were also included. The OSR was to follow him no matter where he went to school in order to ensure a seamless transition in his individual progress. The process was to help teachers be completely up-to-date with the history of their students. Advance knowledge regarding his specific learning disability would have been an invaluable tool as it enabled his teachers to implement strategies that were proven to maximize his learning opportunities.

Despite having this critical information available, it was obvious to us that Steven's new teacher hadn't read the file. Knowing what I do about a teacher's workload, it wasn't completely her fault. I'm sure she was dealing with a host of problems, many of which she was ill-equipped to handle. This angered me because I knew that procedures were in place to insure the OSR file of every "special needs" student transferring into a school was reviewed by the teacher as soon as possible after their arrival. Why had that not been done? Perhaps the principal was at fault, as it was his responsibility to bring it to the teacher's attention. I tried to be as fair as possible. I knew that all too often there were other priorities and situations the principal must deal with, so occasionally a file may not have been reviewed in a timely manner. Also, the sheer logistics of keeping every student interested and engaged was—and still is today—a monumental task. However, as Steven's parents who worried about our son's progress, we were more than frustrated. We felt at that point we were working in a vacuum. The teacher would have been so much better prepared if she had read Steven's file.

> Special education programs and services have come a long way. In Ontario schools today, there are tremendous supports in place to assist children with special needs as well as their teachers. A formal process called Identification, Placement and Review Committee (IPRC), identifies children as "exceptional" and makes decisions about the appropriate programs and services needed to maximize the student's education experience. The process helps students understand their unique needs and how they will be met in the school system. The parents are part of this committee as well as the principal of the school, two staff members, and a special education consultant. The process is successful because it involves the child's parents and the valuable information they can share regarding their child. The IPRC sets the overall framework for the special needs student.
>
> Another major step forward was the creation of the Individual Education Plan (IEP), which is directly tied to the day-to-day teaching of the child. The IEP is reviewed at the beginning of every school term and lays out the short- and long-term expectations for the student, effective strategies for teaching, resources, and any services that may be required to support the student. This document also involves input from the parents and the student whenever possible. Teachers are also supported by adding education assistants when the needs of the child are high, or when the class has several high-needs children.

Steven was nine at this time. His physiotherapy report had been forwarded to the school by KidsAbility as part of their regular assessment. In the report the therapist referred to areas that would improve with therapy, such as improving his range of motion, walking speed, balance, endurance, and posture. "He has difficulty keeping his balance while performing other tasks," the report stated. It also outlined his scoliosis and indicated that he had "difficulty keeping his balance," and that care should be taken not to place him in situations where he had to move quickly or make sudden changes to his gait.

Despite the presence of all this information in Steven's file, his teacher noted in her written evaluation of Steven, "Needs to be reminded to sit up—has a tendency to rest on his desk." When challenged regarding this statement during our parent-teacher interview, the teacher freely admitted she had not seen the physiotherapy report that was part of his OSR. I blew up. I told Steven's teacher that it was painful for us to stand by watching so much valuable time being wasted while the teacher struggled, attempting to use strategies that simply could not work. The stress this situation caused Steven, as well as Linda and me, was counterproductive, and we were very concerned the situation was going to have a negative and lasting impact on Steven's confidence and self-esteem. Had the teacher taken the time to read Steven's file, he would have progressed at a faster pace with more positive results.

In hindsight, I realize that we may have over-reacted a little and could have handled the situation a little differently. We shouldn't have assumed the teacher read the file; rather, we should have requested a meeting with her shortly after Steven arrived at the school to review his file to help her understand Steven's challenges.

WHERE THERE'S A WILL, THERE'S A WAY

Despite these mishaps, at the end of grade one Steven was progressing fairly well academically and was doing well getting around on his own. The special education consultant from KidsAbility, in consultation with his teacher and principal, decided Steven was ready to attend the school that was in our neighborhood. Unfortunately, the bad trend continued in Steven's new school. In grade two we again encountered an insensitive teacher at a parent-teacher interview. We had expected to exchange pleasantries, discuss his habits—both good and bad—and talk about things we could do at home to help with his education. What we heard was shocking. The teacher opened by saying, "Steven is a friendly little boy, but he has a lot of problems! He is very slow, and doesn't pay attention. I don't have the time to spend with him. I am too busy with my regular students and my class!"

To say that I was furious is definitely an understatement. I managed to control my temper and emotions and simply stated, "I thought Steven was a student in your class." Despite what she may have meant to say, what she told us was that Steven was an inconvenience and a distraction to her and the rest of the class. He wasn't part of the class; he was simply "in it." She was clearly unqualified to teach children with special needs. In fairness to her, she obviously had never received adequate special education training, but the lesson was clear. Steven wouldn't always be automatically included. He had to learn how to be part of a group as opposed to being just "in it."

As parents it was up to us to help him navigate that particular minefield. We were fortunate in that Steven, even at that young age, had an indomitable spirit. He just simply figured he belonged. But we had to help him understand in order to truly belong and be accepted, he had to be honest with himself. Although we stressed that he could do anything he wanted to do, and participate in any activity with his friends and classmates, that "right" came with the responsibility of being honest with himself. We told him there were clearly activities that no matter how much he wanted to participate in them, it wouldn't be possible. Steven loved Ice hockey, football, and gymnastics. At first, he accepted our advice and chose to get involved in activities that he felt were within his ability. But then he figured something out. When he couldn't actually take part in an event or sport, he simply became its strongest supporter and best cheer leader. His attitude earned him a lot

> Today many boards of education have "Special Education Advisory Committees" (SEAC) to advocate for children with special needs. The membership of these committees covers a very broad spectrum of stakeholders including members of community organizations and associations representing various disabilities. The role of the committee is to advise the board on all matters related to programs and services that have an impact on children with special needs. Members of these associations bring their concerns to their SEAC representative, who in turn brings the information forward to SEAC committee for discussion. Normally topics discussed at meetings are those that would have an impact on a significant number of children. The children benefit because they and their caretakers are constantly informed of the best services available.

of respect, and eventually, as a cheerleader, he was able to participate in those sports we told him were off limits. What did we know?

Education has come a long way since those days. Teachers now receive better training, and some go on to become specialists in various areas of special education. When it appears the classroom teacher needs help organizing a class with high-needs students, they receive support in the form of education assistants hired specifically to help.

WHAT CAN PARENTS DO?

It would be unfair and inaccurate to suggest that Steven's elementary school experience was entirely negative. In truth, overall he enjoyed his schooling very much during these years. Despite a couple of negative experiences, the majority of the teachers he had throughout grades one to eight were excellent and always willing to help find ways to make it easier for him to learn. In most situations they demonstrated sincere empathy.

But because the possibility exists that Steven's negative experiences are repeatable, I offer you the following list of advice. If you are the parent of a special needs child, this is what I suggest you do to help your child. Remember the earlier you can start these processes, the better:

- ◆ It is important for parents of children with special needs to be actively involved in their child's education from the first day of school.

- ◆ Never assume the school, the principal or your child's teacher is fully informed about your child's disability.

- ◆ Read all the information and notes that are sent home with your child. This is an effective way to monitor activities at the school that your child may be able to participate in. If participation in the activity is possible for your child, be sure to communicate that information with the teacher.

- ◆ If on the other hand participation would be too difficult or unsafe, be sure to explain the reason to your child. This will help reduce the disappointment and more importantly, include your child in the process. The child may not be happy but they will understand.

- Make yourself available to the teacher to discuss your child's progress or difficulties that may surface throughout the year.

- Most boards of education in North America now have equity and inclusion policies that schools must follow. Simply stated, this means that every effort must be made to insure that all school activities such as parties, field trips, or musicals or plays must be open to all children, and accommodations made to ensure participation is possible.

- If your child is in the primary grades, this is a perfect opportunity to educate your child's classmates on his or her disability. Steven was invited to do this by one of his teachers, and it had tremendous results. The children in the class learned about cerebral palsy; they understood why he walked the way he did, and why his arms weren't able to move the same as most children. For Steven, the experience gave him confidence and most importantly, he was accepted by his classmates for who he was, and not a victim of some devastating affliction.

- Finally, make certain the teacher (and school personnel) has a strategy in place with clear plans indicating how your child will be taught, the expectations for the year, and the resources that will be made available to achieve those goals. Most important, make sure you are involved in those discussions.

LEARNING TO NEGOTIATE

In the U.S. and Canada in the 1970's, students with exceptionalities were picked up by smaller school buses. In some situations where it was difficult or impossible for the child to manage getting on and off the bus, a taxicab was used. Once he left the Rotary Centre, Steven's days of being picked up and transported by Driver Bill were over. From this point on, he would be driven to and from school by taxi. We questioned why he couldn't travel with the regular students on the school bus. The reply, at the time, seemed to make sense: the regular school bus simply couldn't accommodate him and it would be very difficult for him to climb onto and off of the bus every day. What they really meant was that he was too slow and that he would hold the bus up too long as he climbed on and off with his crutches.

Like everything else he had endured in his short life, he met all kinds of challenges when it came to his cab drivers. Both Linda and I cringed every morning as we waited anxiously to see what type of personality would show up in the driveway. There were those who simply did their job, not getting involved with the children or even participating in conversation; for them the children were simply another fare. There were others that left us feeling concerned for Steven's well-being. In those days, they didn't have laws in place preventing drivers from smoking while customers were in their cab. Leaving the window open while they puffed away was of little help to those poor souls riding in the back seat. One can only imagine the air quality during inclement weather or in the winter when the windows had to remain closed.

There was also the occasional driver who did not like to drive children with disabilities because they took a little extra time to get settled into their seats. Usually the school board designed pickups so the cab could accommodate at least two children at a time, but some drivers openly complained about how much money they were losing because of all the time it took to transport disabled children.

Every evening Steven would tell us about his day and his experiences in the cab. He told us about impolite drivers, and sometimes he would proudly repeat an assortment of new words he had heard that day. We were appalled, but instead of reprimanding him for cursing like a sailor, we explained to him that some drivers were unhappy about taking students to school because they thought they were losing opportunities to pick up other customers. It was hard for Steven to understand that it wasn't him personally who was upsetting the driver. Our advice was to respect the driver, behave, and be polite at all times—no matter how blue the air would get. We made sure he understood how important

THE WORST OF TIMES AND THE BEST OF TIMES

it was to respect his elders. He soon found out that our advice was sound and that it was the best approach to take, as he often witnessed the frustration of other special needs students responding to various negative situations. By taking the high road, he bypassed a lot of personal frustration and avoided confrontation.

In time, Steven began to report that his daily trips to and from school were "okay," and that some of the bad drivers he had experienced in the past were now treating him civilly and were even initiating conversations with him. He was learning how to deal with the situation on his own. On a few occasions, however, his treatment was so insensitive we felt the need to intervene. If we found a situation was escalating, or we were concerned about Steven's welfare, we would discuss the situation and the specific driver with the Special Education Department at the school board. We never suggested a driver be reprimanded, choosing instead to suggest that the taxi company consider transferring the driver off the school pickups.

Not every experience with the taxi drivers was bad; Steven was very lucky throughout his time at school to have drivers who were caring and friendly. I recall a driver by the name of Joe who must have truly loved his job. He was always patient with Steven and never complained when he was a little tardy either at home or at the end of the school day. He took a personal interest in Steven, at times reporting directly to us if he suspected something was wrong. In the morning he would park in the driveway and wait patiently, or he would ring the doorbell and help Steven out to the car. He smoked cigars but rarely smoked when the kids were in the cab. Joe had a caring attitude and was always sensitive to the well-being of the children. He was also funny, teasing the kids when the opportunity presented itself.

Some drivers would assist the kids by carrying their books to the cab for them at the end of the day; others simply engaged in small talk. The important thing for us was that they demonstrated sensitivity and respect for the children, which in turn made our lives a lot less stressful as well.

A VERY SPECIAL SUMMER CAMP

The winter Steven celebrated his ninth birthday, we took him to one of his regular evaluation sessions at the Rotary Centre. During the conversation, his therapists recommended we consider applying to send Steven to Woodeden, a summer camp for the physically challenged, located near London, Ontario, and sponsored by the Canadian Easter Seals Society. We didn't know much about the camp, or the Canadian Easter Seals Association; we had many questions to ask. Steven had never been away without his family before, so this would definitely be a new experience for us all. However, the most important benefit was the chance for him to be like many other kids his age by attending a summer camp. We needed time to think about it and discuss it before we made our decision. As we left the center with the information they provided about the camp and the association, as well as the application form, their parting words were, "Don't wait too long. The camp has a limited number of spaces available and they go very fast."

Steven was excited and eager to go to the camp; he couldn't understand why we didn't just fill out the papers then and there. Although it seemed like a terrific opportunity, we still wanted to mull it over and make sure Steven clearly understood the camp lasted two weeks and was a considerable distance from home so he couldn't change his mind once he was there. A couple of days later, I dropped the application forms off at the center. We had decided this was an outstanding opportunity for Steven that may not be available again in the future. All the reports we read and the references we received on Woodeden painted a glowing picture of a summer camp that was perfect for any child with physical disabilities. A couple weeks later we received his acceptance letter.

It seemed like an eternity for Steven as the days leading up to summer vacation went by. Finally the day arrived to take him to his first summer camp. He was so excited he couldn't sleep the night before.

During the drive to London, Linda and I quietly talked about the "what if" factor. What if he changed his mind and didn't want to stay? We envisioned him crying and clinging to us, begging us not to leave him there alone. After a considerably long drive, we arrived at the entrance to the camp. It was a magnificent secluded setting on more than one hundred acres within a forest overlooking the Thames River.

As we unloaded Steven's luggage and wheelchair from the car, we avoided eye contact with him so he wouldn't break down. Imagine our shock and disappointment when he eagerly sat in the wheelchair and bolted down the lane to meet up with the other kids. He was ecstatic. A camp councilor introduced himself to us and explained what would be going on for the campers over the next two weeks. It sounded like so much fun Linda and I thought perhaps we should stay with him.

The goal of the camp was to give children with a variety of disabilities and challenges the opportunity to experience all the fun things other kids have the chance to experience at a summer camp. They would be with their peers so they would not feel "different" and could enjoy the experience without competing. Their health and safety was assured by a staff of more than sixty including four live-in nurses.

> **Every child with physical or intellectual challenges should have the same opportunities as other children. This includes the fun of attending a summer camp. Summer camp can give them a brief respite from their challenge, an opportunity not to be different.**
>
> **There are many organizations such as Easter Seals that operate camps that cater to children with various disabilities. They provide programs that allow the child to experience new things, make new friends, and develop leadership skills. The camp experience can also help the child learn vital life skills such as making good choices.**
>
> **The experience also helps the child develop independence, self-confidence, and an acceptance of "who they are", and what they are capable of achieving. I strongly recommend every parent try to give their child a chance to attend a summer camp. Most organizations have programs that provide financial assistance to families that may otherwise be unable to afford to send their child.**

Throughout the next two weeks they would have a chance to swim, go sailing, play basketball and sledge hockey, and participate in arts and crafts such as pottery. One outstanding feature was a tree house that was fully accessible and used for overnight "sleep-outs" and campfires.

Parents were invited to visit the camp and their child on the second weekend for a surprise presentation. We thought, "Okay, he's had a full week from us. By now he will definitely be ready to come home!" We prepared ourselves for the scene that might unfold because we had convinced ourselves that two weeks may have been a little too much for his first time.

When we arrived and parked the car, Steven was already there waiting. He was so excited to see us—but the expected request for an immediate trip home never materialized. He couldn't stop talking about the previous week and all the activities he had participated in. He introduced us to all his new friends that must have been just about every other boy and girl in the camp.

The surprise presentation was a play the kids put together with every camper having a part to play. Parents thoroughly enjoyed the program; many laughs and a few tears were shed that day. They were so proud of themselves, and we were so happy to see the difference Woodeden was making in their lives.

At the end of the day, it was time for parents to leave again. It was obvious to all of us that our presence was keeping the campers from having their fun. We recognized that it was us who were having the hard time being separated from him, but we also knew that while we were sad to leave him again, we were happy beyond words with the incredible experience this was for him and all the other children with challenges.

Steven enjoyed the Woodeden adventure so much he returned the following year to re-acquaint himself with his old friends. It had a lifelong impact on him because it gave him and his friends the chance to try new things without competing with other children in a regular camp setting.

EAGER TO PARTICIPATE

Steven and his brothers were a few years apart in age so they didn't really spend a lot of time playing together. David, the eldest, was seven years older than Steven, and Scott was four years older. They love their brother, and when he was younger, they wanted to protect him but, as we had so carefully taught them, it was important to let Steven be himself. His oldest brother, David, recalls everyone's favorite side of Steven, the humorous side. "He always seemed to find a way to laugh at himself, to make light of an embarrassing situation. We always treated him like the typical younger brother—teased him, tormented him, and constantly reminded him he was a pain in the neck. We really never saw him as "handicapped." That was okay for Scott and me, but we drew the line at others picking on him. I found it upsetting when others stared at him when we were out together. During those times when Steven was in a wheelchair, we would make a game of getting from one place to another in the shortest period of time possible, meaning we would tilt the chair back on the rear wheels, stand on the back, and propel ourselves past everyone. Since we didn't appear to have a lot of control of our vehicle, people usually parted as quickly as they could. I remember those times he had surgery; we felt helpless because there was nothing we could do to ease his pain or make him feel comfortable."

Scott remembered on a cold winter day when all three brothers somehow found themselves at home together without plans with friends—an unusual occurrence for the older boys. It was around the Christmas holiday and, "we thought it would be fun to go to NCR (NCR operated a large manufacturing facility close to our home) to ride our toboggan. So we bundled up and proceeded to strike out for the hill. It was cold and windy, and a good hike when you consider we had Steven with us. We were only outside for about half an hour when Steven began to complain that he was really cold. Dave and I didn't realize that when Steven gets really cold his muscles tighten up causing them to become spastic and painful for him. When I say tighten up, I mean like rigor mortis! By the time we realized how serious it was, it was too late. We had to get home as quickly as we could before it got worse. You have to remember, we were brothers, so at the time, we found this somewhat amusing and so did Steven. We put Steven on the toboggan and headed toward home running as fast as we could, taking turns pulling. When we finally got home, we were completely exhausted, and it took Steven a couple hours to thaw out enough to get around on his own. It was, all things considered, a good day because it wasn't very often the three of us did something together. I think, other than the pain, Steven would agree."

Steven was a child who seemed to ignore danger, or perhaps he felt nothing serious would ever happen to him if he tried to take part in the same activities as his brothers or friends from around the neighborhood. During the winter he would bundle up, grab a hockey stick, and head out to the street for a game of road hockey. It was quite a site; he never stood up straight, and he fell a lot. He always claimed it was the ice and that he had slipped. His hockey stick, more times than not, gave him support and balance. Even though he was always the last person chosen for a team, he was overjoyed that he could play. When he got tired, he would play in goal and occasionally even made a few saves. His style always provided a certain amount of humor. I still recall the image of this kid using a goalie stick as a replacement for his crutches flailing away wildly at thin air whenever the puck came anywhere close to him. For him, the game was real, and he was in it—just like all the others. He would be thoroughly focused on stopping the puck at any cost, and that focus was clearly evident by the look of determination on his face. He would laugh right along with his friends when he would lose his balance and awkwardly fall to the road, simultaneously making an outstanding save.

His eagerness to participate in sports extended to his school as well. He loved to attend gym class and take part in as many of the physical activities as he could. When he got home at night he would be filled with excitement, telling us every detail about the fun he had at school playing various sports. Some teachers actually encouraged him to try and do whatever he could while unfortunately others would have him sit on the sidelines and watch. Their insensitivity seemed to be based more on ignorance of his disability than real concern for his well-being. As Steven grew older, I realized as I had with his learning challenges that I had to "educate" his teachers on what he could and couldn't do physically.

I recall speaking to one of his teachers and suggesting that it was okay with Steven's mother and me if he was allowed to participate in activities like basketball, floor hockey, or even volleyball. Steven wasn't made of glass, I explained. If he fell, he wasn't going to break, and even if he did fall, his injuries would not be any worse than any other child in the class. My recommendation was to allow Steven to decide for himself if an activity was too dangerous or difficult. The teacher seemed a bit shocked at first. I have downplayed the negative or shocked reactions people had, and still have, toward Steven. I don't like to dwell on it, but this teacher reminded me of how the world views people with exceptionalities. We're always, unfortunately, a bit surprised when someone doesn't quite look like us or even sound like us. But part of my role as a parent, I realized early on, was to help Steven and others see past the physical challenges, and see the boy who was willing to try anything. He was a boy after all, and that's what boys do!

We knew it sometimes bothered Steven that he couldn't keep up with his friends and classmates, but we encouraged him to just do the best he could. Even though he couldn't keep up, his friends admired his determination and willingness to try. They seemed to provide the encouragement he really needed, the kind that came from friends who cared. It started building strong character in him very early in life.

Dr. Norman Vincent Peale once wrote, "It's always too soon to quit." We tried to instill in Steven the attitude that no matter how bad things seemed to be, he should never stop trying. We would tell him the secret: "Want something so bad you can't give up." Each one of our boys received the same advice: when things are so bad it seems like there is no solution, make some breathing room by taking a step back, and then try again. Usually this intermission from the problem helps clear the cobwebs and allows a potential plan of action to surface.

TRIUMPH OVER CHALLENGES

There were times when our hearts would ache for the pain Steven was feeling when he wasn't given the chance to be "normal" like his friends. On one occasion his elementary school was having their annual track and field meet. It was a big event. Students could win medals when they finished in the top three positions as well as for participation. The competitions had lasted well into the afternoon, everything from broad jumping to races. Steven waited patiently throughout the entire day, cheering on his classmates and helping with various events to keep the participants focused. Finally when it was his turn to take part, he was told by the teacher that they had run out of time and that he couldn't complete his event. "You don't have to compete today, Steven. We don't have any more time; but don't worry we have a medal for you anyway," the teacher said.

I will never forget how proud I was of him when he told me his response to the teacher, "I don't want the medal if I didn't compete like the others."

Years later he explained to us that taking the medal would not have been right; he felt he didn't earn it so it didn't hold any meaning for him. Steven's comment didn't seem to have any effect on the teacher at the time, but I am sure when he had time to reflect, he would have realized that his gesture was patronizing and more important, I hope he realized what a gift Steven gave him that day by refusing.

It's always interesting to look back on what happened in our children's lives. I remember the hardships, but I rejoice in the triumphs. For every negative experience Steven had in terms of his physical disability, it was countered with something positive, even amazing. Steven had one particular teacher that was clearly ahead of his time. Every year, the school held an event they called the Cross Canada Run. Each student in the school who wished to participate was allowed to take part. The event involved running around the block and back to the school, a distance of one kilometer. As the total number of kilometers added up, they would be applied to a map of Canada. The goal was not only to involve the students in physical activity but also to teach them about their country as the accumulated distances traversed from one coast to the other.

Steven talked about this event for weeks; he was excited about proving to everyone that he could do it. We were more concerned about how badly he would feel if he was told he couldn't participate. The day he indicated to the teacher that he intended to participate, he was as surprised as we were when his teacher, Mr. Kearns, gave him his approval.

The only conditions were that he had to have our permission, he had to be sure it wasn't going to be too difficult, and he had to promise that if he felt too tired, or was too sore, he would drop out. Steven enthusiastically agreed. He went on to complete the race in record time. The record wasn't for the fastest time, I believe it was for the slowest—but he did it! The most amazing part of this story was that Mr. Kearns ran the entire race with him. What an incredible display of support and compassion. He made Steven feel like he was finally one of the boys.

We have never forgotten that day. Mr. Kearns was a teacher in the true sense of the word. "This project was really significant to me because there was never any question about my participation," Steven said. "He—Mr. Kearns—let me be part of it. I remember how great it felt to have a sense of accomplishment and to be pushed to my own limits every day. There were consequences, mostly related to physical issues, but I would do it again if I ever had the opportunity."

Fortunately, the positive experiences throughout his elementary and secondary school life far outweighed the number of negative incidents with teachers. As I said in the beginning of this chapter, attitudes toward the teaching of exceptional children were changing quickly in the seventies and eighties. Enhanced programming, increased access to resources, and dedicated teaching professionals were making the learning experience more meaningful and effective for the children. Special education programs and services have made significant advances since the early years when Steven attended his first regular school class.

Good teachers worked with Steven to help him understand the various subjects in class; they took the time to make sure he didn't fall behind or become frustrated and just give up. Every now and then, a great teacher would come along. This individual would not only treat him the same as the other children in the class, he or she would challenge him to do more and prove to himself that he could do much better if he really tried.

Another principle we tried to help Steven understand was that when he was attempting a new skill or trying to learn a new lesson at school, to not be upset if he wasn't successful on the first or second attempt. Sometimes, failure can be a good thing as we learn and profit from our mistakes. It would upset us when someone would point out his mistakes and tell him it was okay, suggesting that he could try something different—or easier. How would it be possible for him to learn and grow if he was taught that it is acceptable to fail and not learn from his mistakes? Throughout his childhood we focused more on things he could do rather than talking about the things he could not do. Our guidance helped as he never approached anything with an "escape excuse" but rather the confidence he could do it. He took that advice and used it to his advantage—often.

LEARNING WHEN TO QUIT

One of the hardest lessons Steven had to learn, though, was when to give up no matter how hard he tried to succeed. The Air Cadet Corps was one of those times. In Ingersol, Ontario I have two good friends, Paul Tambeau, and his wife, Sharon. Paul was a group Commanding Officer for the Region in the Air Cadet movement when Steven was young and Sharon was the Commanding Officer of the Air Cadet Corps Steven was in. I was visiting them a while back. We struck up a conversation about the Air Cadets while we were watching the Corps drill.

While observing a member of the Corps that has cerebral palsy, Paul couldn't help but remember his experience with Steven: "He was born at a time when conditions like cerebral palsy prevented people like Steven from being totally integrated into mainstream society." Paul was referring to the attempt Steven made to join and be active in a local Cadet Corps. Steven was intrigued by the opportunities it would provide him, like taking part in activities with his friends, belonging to an organization, and committing to the rigors of actively participating in a wide variety of events and activities. The Cadet Corps in the beginning was very reluctant to allow him to join and employed many excuses to discourage him from applying. He would have great difficulty marching, the activities they had would be too physically demanding, and a career in the military in later years would be out of the question. Eventually he wore them down; he was determined he could do it.

THE WORST OF TIMES AND THE BEST OF TIMES

I remember him coming home with his uniform. He was so proud of himself; he couldn't stop talking about all the things he was going to be doing. During the first few weeks everything seemed to be going smoothly, but after that we started to notice he wasn't so enthusiastic anymore. He never complained, but I knew something was wrong. The last event he participated in was a tag day, where he was required to spend a few hours on his feet selling tags in support of the air cadet squadron. Standing on his feet for long hours was extremely tiring and painful for him, but he endured the pain to prove to his friends as well as to the officers that he was a capable cadet and was contributing. However, instead of acknowledging his determination and enthusiasm with a simple "well done," he was counseled to consider leaving the Corps. They told him it wasn't working out and that it was obviously too difficult for him.

While we viewed their attitude as discriminating and intolerant, he didn't want to cause problems in the Corps, so he decided to quit. Steven wasn't a quitter, but in his heart he felt it was the right thing to do. To the very end, despite the way he was treated, he respected the organization and settled for accepting the situation as just another minor setback.

Paul said, "I've always thought of Steven as somewhat easy going, tending to take things in stride (especially his physical condition), thoughtful and yet very determined. We all know how society has changed in the last few decades with respect to access for people with special needs. To Steven's credit, he dealt with the challenges mostly

> Today, things are much different in many organizations, including military cadet corps. Young people with various disabilities are not prevented or discouraged from joining and participating in the variety of programs offered. Accommodations are made for those that are physically challenged that are both inclusive and inviting. The focus of the cadet corps is to help young boys and girls become better citizens, discipline, and to experience the military. Although many of the cadets go on to joining the regular armed forces after graduation, it isn't the main focus of the cadet corps.

on his own without the help of his family and friends. No one can know what it's like to deal with the challenges Steven and all the "Stevens" face on a daily basis; only they can, and only their parents can know what you deal with raising a child with special needs."

CREATIVE DAYDREAMING

More than anything else Steven believed in himself. It's something we fostered in him, most definitely, but he has a core of strength that is remarkable. But here's the shocking thing we both had to learn. While I discovered over the years a strong sense of self-belief is a great quality to have, in the end it isn't enough. If Steven's belief wasn't backed up by action, he would never have achieved his goals.

So one of the lessons I'm most proud of teaching Steven is learning how to act on his belief. From a very early age, we taught him how to pretend he had already accomplished his goals. I called it "creative daydreaming." We strongly subscribe to the principle that if you could imagine achieving your goal, somehow your mind would help you find the means to do it. There have been several books written on this topic referring to it as "imaging" or "visualization." Any child or adult with challenges absolutely needs to believe in themselves and their potential, or their battle will be a very tough one, and the best way to tap into that belief is through this "creative daydreaming."

Steven put his "creative daydreaming" to use many times during his therapy sessions, particularly after several operations on his legs. Repeated surgery left him with very little muscle tone; in fact his left leg was quite thin with only a small amount of muscle remaining. After repeated surgery that involved cutting the tendons on that leg, it began to "atrophy" or waste away because it no longer was able to develop naturally. The end result was that walking became increasingly challenging for him. I often marveled how he kept doing it but he never succumbed to a wheelchair. He was determined to remain independent.

We'll never forget what he told us following one of his therapy sessions. He had just recently had his body cast removed after hip surgery.

THE WORST OF TIMES AND THE BEST OF TIMES

It was one of those depressing days for him when everything he tried had failed. He just couldn't make his legs function properly and walking even a few steps seemed impossible. Tired and frustrated he turned to Linda and me and simply said, "I'm not going to let this beat me!" It made me cry and then laugh with pride.

That has always been my Steven. He always wrote off those bad days with the attitude, "tomorrow will be better!" In terms of therapy, many would have given up, surrendering to the enduring pain. However, giving up was never an option. Steven was determined and focused on the task of learning to walk again.

Many years ago, Dr. Norman Vincent Peale, in his book *You Can If You Think You Can*, talks about the power of having a strong belief—that you can reach your goals if you believe and never give up. Many people since Dr. Peale have picked up on that idea. I made a point of instilling that concept in Steven when he was a little boy. But I have always wondered how much of it he already knew.

CHAPTER FOUR

Friends, Basketball, and Falling Down Stairs

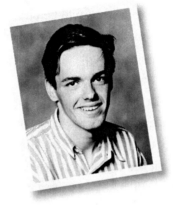

People become really quite remarkable when they start thinking that they can do things. When they believe in themselves they have the first secret of success.

Norman Vincent Peale

When Steven graduated from grade eight, we were so proud of him. His determination and positive attitude continued to blossom, and while we worried about the dramatic changes he might face in the transition from elementary school to high school, Steven couldn't wait. We thought of a hundred things to fret about. How would he be able to change classes and be on time when the next period started? How would he fit in with the other students? Could he handle the pressures of high school and the course material? Suddenly we remembered: didn't we worry about exactly the same things when our other two boys entered secondary school?

When Steven was a youngster, we had often been told to not count on Steven being able to attend high school. Linda and I always kept that little negative tidbit a secret from Steven. We wanted him to make that decision for himself—not some therapist working with the law of averages. High school was simply the necessary next step in Steven's education and maturation. Linda and I were apprehensive but this is what we had hoped for him. And Steven being Steven, we knew he would make the best of it and enjoy the experience.

BUCKING THE ODDS

The recommendation of his elementary schools' teachers and principal, supported by his therapists, was that Steven should attend an accessible school where elevators were available or at least where his classes would be on the main floor. The school they thought appropriate would also have several other youngsters with a variety of physical challenges so he wouldn't feel "alone."

Of course, Steven had other ideas.

While these discussions concerning his schooling were going on between his therapists and us, Steven was doing a little research of his own. He discovered that most of his close friends were attending Bluevale Collegiate, only a five-minute drive from our home. When we told him our thoughts, he politely told us that he had made up his mind that he was going to Bluevale. We made sure that he understood the challenges he would face. He was okay with all of them.

> Therapists, teachers, doctors, any caregiver, are well meaning, but sometimes they will give parents and their children limiting ideas and beliefs about the child. One mom told me about her daughter's first grade teacher who cautioned her that her daughter's IQ was a bit low so "don't expect too much." The mother never told the child who went on to not only graduate college Magna Cum Laude but completed her Ph.D. That "challenged" child is a twice-published author and very successful business owner. Be cautious of what you let your child hear from his or her caregivers, and always encourage your child to strive for their very best, whatever that best may be.

"I remember pushing mom and dad to let me to go to Bluevale. I knew it had lots of steps and in some ways wasn't accessible but that didn't matter to me. Right from the time I had my first tour of the school until I graduated a few years later, it was one of the most important places and times in my life. My friends were going there and it had the best environment. There was always so much energy, and everyone was encouraged to get involved."

It didn't take very long before he put all our fears to rest. He had found his niche. He was making friends and participating in virtually every activity the school would allow. One afternoon he arrived home and proudly announced he was going to try out for the upcoming musical production. We weren't quite sure how to respond to this. After all, we were the supportive parents who spent years helping him build his self-confidence and convincing him to try anything he felt he was capable of doing. Not once did he even consider that he might fail. His goal was to be part of it; he didn't care what role he would play, as long as he was involved.

Steven secured a role with the technical crew responsible for the lighting. He was possibly the hardest working, most committed member in the production. There wasn't anything he wouldn't do or attempt to do. Prior to the start of the show's opening night, Linda and I spoke to his drama teacher for a few minutes; we were interested in hearing how Steven fared in his first school musical production. The teacher told us, "I've never seen a student work so hard to prove himself." She then confided, "We had to say no to him a few times because he literally volunteered for everything!" However, the anecdote that took our breath away went something like this: One afternoon while rehearsals were going on, there was a request to relocate overhead lighting—a job for the technical lighting crew. Of course, boys will be boys, and he insisted he could do the same work as the rest of his crew. Without a moment's hesitation, Steven proceeded to make his way out on the cat-walk high above the stage to make the necessary adjustment. By the time reality set in, it was too late and he was precariously crawling along the metal frame. Everyone remained calm and pretended not to panic, but in the back of their minds they envisioned him plummeting to the ground at any moment. Somehow, miraculously, he pulled it off, making the required lighting adjustment and returning safely to the floor below.

By the end of the week, most of the teachers at the school were aware of his escapade. Opinions varied, ranging from disbelief to "Can you imagine what would have happened if he fell and was seriously injured—or worse?" There were also feelings of extreme admiration for his team-player attitude and the fact that he was willing to try anything.

A TURNING POINT

The high school experience, although feared by us, became a turning point in Steven's life. He immediately took to the relatively unstructured environment and thrived on it. In a sense, it was therapeutic because he was forced to walk from one class to the next at the end of each period giving him much needed exercise and stretching. It was also easier for him to concentrate because the classes were only forty minutes long. The time between classes allowed him a few minutes to recharge. Most importantly, he began to associate with many new students although engaging new friends never seemed to be an issue with him. Linda and I noticed him change over time; his self-confidence increased. He wanted to join everything but found a passion in the sports programs at the school, particularly basketball. Steven had developed a passion for basketball a couple of summers earlier, during one of our family vacations to Florida, and in his inimitable way, he found a way to act on that passion.

> It is crucial that you encourage your child to participate in as many activities as he or she is capable of. It continually fosters that all-important self-confidence, and both the child and those around him/her learn how to handle themselves in varied situations.

"The single most important impact of high school on me was my involvement in the junior and senior boys' basketball programs," Steven declared. "For the first time in my life I was part of a team, not as a player but as team manager. I supported both teams with scorekeeping and operating the time clocks for the home and away games. I traveled with the team and learned a lot about teamwork, about the sport of basketball, and many other important things. I have some unforgettable memories like winning the championship. The guys were always there for each other," Steven said.

HANDLING ADVERSITY

Surgery and Steven were no strangers. As a young child, Steven endured several painful operations as a result of his muscles and ligaments not handling the natural growth. This is very common with cerebral palsy. We were very fortunate to have an excellent orthopedic surgeon recommended to us through the Rotary Centre. Dr. James Israel evaluated and consulted on Steven's case as well as on many of the Rotary children for several years. Dr. Israel got to know all of the children on his caseload at the center personally taking an interest in their progress and helping families make the best of surgical situations. He was truly a blessing, and I am pleased to say that the good doctor went on to become the chief of medical staff at the Grand River Hospital in Kitchener, Ontario.

Whenever surgery was deemed necessary for Steven, Dr. Israel would coordinate the details. When he was in high school, Steven had to have surgery on his knee to correct the rotation that was causing him a lot of pain and hindered his ability to walk. The procedure was required because of the impact of earlier surgeries that cut tendons and muscles to allow for growth. The lack of muscle and tendon resulted in his leg turning inward from constantly putting pressure on it while walking.

Whenever he had to go through one of his operations, it was quite stressful for everyone in the family, particularly for Linda and me. The hospital in Hamilton was more than an hour away from our home, and usually the duration of his stay averaged one to two weeks. We couldn't be with him as much as we wanted and that bothered us, but Steven handled each occasion with a remarkable attitude. The nurses would constantly comment on how he happily chatted with them from the moment he woke up in the morning until he went to bed at night.

Steven became a student of medical procedures. By the time he left the hospital for home, he would know the medical term for every muscle, tendon, and joint affected by his surgery. Hospital staff said he was like a sponge, absorbing every detail of his procedure no matter how minor. At times he was uncomfortable but he never asked for medication unless he could no longer tolerate the pain. What was always most remarkable to me, however, was the big part he played in helping other patients keep the pain off their minds. We saw it when we visited, and his doctors and nurses always made sure we knew what was going on.

Prior to the surgery Dr. Israel would meet with Linda and me as well as Steven to discuss the scope of the surgery and what to expect post-op. Since some of the surgical procedures Steven went through were very complex, they were performed at McMaster University Medical Centre in Hamilton, Ontario. But the therapy and follow-up took place in Kitchener with one follow-up appointment with the surgeon in Hamilton. Dr. Israel would also make it clear to Steven what he could expect in the way of results and the amount of therapy that would be required during the recovery stage. Therapy was the part Steven hated; as did all children having similar procedures, it was usually very uncomfortable and almost always painful. However despite the lengthy recovery and rehabilitation period, he returned to school optimistic and determined to take part in every possible activity.

JUST ANOTHER ONE OF THE GUYS

Steven was fearless, that's for certain. He also had a knack for just being "one of the guys." He never let his disability get in the way of him participating, even when the pranks involved him. One afternoon we received a call from the school to inform us there had been a little "accident" involving Steven, but not to worry, that he was okay. Apparently what had happened was that three of his friends had decided to carry him up to the second floor so he could remain with his regular class. At the time, he had just returned to school following surgery and was confined to a wheelchair for a few weeks. Everything was going according to plan when one of the boys lost his balance and his grip on the wheelchair sending Steven tumbling down the flight of stairs. He was pretty sore, sporting a few bruises, but without any serious damage. The vice principal of the school wasn't very amused and shared his views with Steven's three "helpers." Of course, he was quite correct in his concerns. The results could have been tragic. All four boys learned a lesson that day, and the dangerous practice of carrying Steven up the stairs in a wheelchair came to an abrupt end.

All shenanigans aside, Steven's "can do" spirit didn't go unnoticed. The high school activity director, George Hunsberger, at the time saw something in Steven that went beyond his disabilities. He saw the impact he had on others and decided to capitalize on it. "I got to know Steven when he was in grade nine," George remembered. "I'm not sure why, but Steven ended up being the scorekeeper and timer for the junior boys' basketball team that I coached. I approached him, rather than waiting for the annual gaggle of female grade nine students who inevitably wanted to volunteer for the job just to be around the boys.

"My impression of Steven after watching him for the first few weeks of the school year was that here was a kid with severe physical limitations, often in severe pain, but who never complained! If he was like that during every school day, maybe he would radiate those same positive vibes in a team setting during our thirty games, sixty practices, numerous bus rides, and navigation in and out of different schools and tournaments. He was even better than that! He did inspire the team, but more important, he became a part of it. We had some talented basketball players during those two years before Steven moved up to the senior setting to stay with 'his team.' They just loved having Steven around. They would kid him, tease him gently, and treat him just like any other member of the team." During Steven's time at Bluevale Collegiate, George became Steven's mentor and friend, and they have remained close over the years.

Doros Theodosiou, one of Steven's teammates and friends from his high school days, shared George's thoughts. "That particular group of basketball players back then was a very special group, and Steven was part of it. We never looked at Steven as someone with a disability, but rather part of the team. When I think back to the impression Steven left with me, it was that he never looked at himself as someone with a disability. He never shied away from doing what he thought someone without a disability could do like being the manager of a basketball team. Regardless of what Coach Hunsberger or a player asked of him, he always did it. Confidence was a big part of Steven as he always felt comfortable with us and we felt the same with him. I think many parents of children with disabilities unfortunately shy away from getting their kids involved with the mainstream, be it sports or other outlets. Looking back I am convinced getting [these kids] involved early in life is a big factor."

Steven had no shortage of close friends in high school. His disability was hardly ever a factor as he participated in everything he possibly could. He was very attentive, absorbing the details of every conversation. He was also a good listener, often providing the shoulder to cry on or administering advice when called upon. He went to dances; most times forgetting he was challenged. I don't make that comment flippantly. I remember driving him to school one morning, as he was running late, but when we arrived at the school he realized he had forgotten his crutches. Naturally, I couldn't resist asking the obvious question, "How could someone with cerebral palsy, who has walked with crutches every day for most of his life, forget his crutches?" It was a rhetorical question at the time, and we still laugh about it to this day.

THE SOCIAL ANIMAL

Steven has always had one of those magnetic personalities that seem to captivate everyone around him. He was the favorite uncle—he loves his nieces and they, him. David's daughters, Kirstie and Taylor, are now attending university high school respectively. Scott's kids, Alyssa and Kyle, are in high school. Since each of these girls has been able to talk, they have been very close to Steven. He has always been interested in what's going on in their lives and somehow is able to communicate on virtually any topic they want to discuss. At family gatherings it isn't uncommon for all of them to steal away into the basement to listen to music on the computer or, as Steven would say, "just hang out." Many times Steven would be their source of entertainment as he would lose his balance, trip over someone's feet, show up characteristically late, or polish off two and three helpings of his mother's cooking. Treating him just like they treated each other seemed to come naturally. Linda and I are sure a lot of their attitude came from David and Scott who formed the original support team for Steven.

Steven was definitely a "guy's guy," but he was also very charming with the girls. Even when he was young, he would always have a bunch of girls for friends. But in the back of our minds, Linda and I worried about Steven's transition to high school. This was the age teenagers begin to take an active interest in the opposite sex. All teens, whether or not they have a disability, begin to think about dating and having a girlfriend or boyfriend. The problem arises when it comes to the "going out on a date" part. Most of the time teens with a disability are not as mobile as their friends, and of course, the fear of rejection is huge. Our concern was the impact rejection would have on him. Would it set him back and destroy his self-confidence? Would it change his attitude about himself and how he lived with his challenge? Every parent of a child with a disability worries about the age of self-discovery.

Fortunately for us, and I suppose for Steven, most of his classmates and friends hung out in groups and dating never was an issue. On occasion he would ask a girl to a dance, and we were all pleasantly surprised when she accepted. In those situations we would usually drive him to the dance and the two of them would meet there. It must have cramped his style, but we also picked him up and drove his date home as well. He never really got upset when he was turned down. I guess he saw the same thing happened to his friends, so it seemed normal.

Brandy Duchesne-Martin, Steven's long-time friend from his earlier years at the Rotary Centre, didn't attend the same high school but they remained friends over the years. About their friendship, Brandy says, "I have known Steven for such a long time. Our friendship was such a strong support for me, particularly during my teenage and early adult years. Thinking back on our friendship during our younger years, what I remember and love most about Steven is his determination, passion for life, compassion for others, and his inner strength. He was always

FRIENDS, BASKETBALL, AND FALLING DOWN STAIRS

talking about his plans for the future and his plan to get there. He also talked about how much he loved his work—no matter what sort—voluntary or otherwise, he was committed with his energy, heart, and drive. He always expressed such love and loyalty to his family and friends and didn't ever neglect to tell us how important we were to him. He would always say he wanted to do important things—to be "someone"—and to know that what he did or was doing would make an impact, that it would be important to people and have a positive effect on their lives and make a difference." Brandy is another huge success story. She went on to graduate from the University of Waterloo and married James Martin. They now have a beautiful little daughter, Elise.

Linda and I should have never worried about Steven's transition to high school. Steven was—and still is—the ultimate social animal. Linda and I always encouraged him to step boldly into the world, to not ever be ashamed of his disabilities. He never was. Instead, he seized every opportunity he could, talking to just about anyone who would listen. He loved to feel he didn't have limits, offering to help in any situation he could. Money was never a consideration; he just wanted to be part of something.

We have lived close to a shopping mall for many years, so Steven had plenty of opportunity to spend time meeting people and making friends in a variety of the retail stores—something he later turned into employment opportunities. One of the individuals he met was Nick Renda, the manager of the Joggers store. Steven was fifteen at the time, too young to apply for a job, but not too young to develop an affinity to the retail business. Nick's first impression of Steven was that he would not let anything slow him down: "I've always known Steve to go after whatever he wanted. He would never talk about his disability. It was almost as if he wasn't even aware he had one. He was a very smart and positive person. The one thing I will always remember is when he used to come into the store to say hello to everyone and strike up a conversation. He would never talk about himself or his day; he only wanted to hear about how our day had been. He would then proceed to help us place shoes that were left lying around back on the wall display. It was almost like he worked there. His personality and demeanor was always positive and he was always very happy." In the years ahead, Nick became a very close friend and role model for Steven. He would come to the house to pick up Steven to take in a movie, or go to a restaurant, or just hang out. Steven still is able to make friends, male and female, whenever and wherever he is.

WHO ME, DISABLED?

While our boys were students, our family had the good fortune to participate in numerous youth-exchange programs. We learned of the exchange student program through the Rotary Club. We had met a wonderful Japanese student through the Rotary Youth Exchange Program. Her name was Yumi Hirakawa, and while she wasn't our exchange daughter, she became part of the family during the year she spent in the States. Yumi has remained a part of our family for almost twenty years. When she arrived, she was a frightened but very friendly and personable teenager from Gyoda, Japan. Yumi spent many weekends with us, participated in countless family get-togethers including Christmas and Thanksgiving, and traveled with us to Florida where she and Steven sang karaoke one evening to a very enthusiastic audience response. We were aware of Steven's vocal talent, but we had never heard Yumi sing. It was incredible!

When I wrote and asked her to share her memories of Steven, Yumi wrote back, "I've known Steve since he was a teenager. He is always very friendly to everyone and very positive about his life. His parents have hosted exchange students from all over the world, and watching him I saw he always treated everyone with respect and a kind heart. It's hard to imagine his father writing a book about his life for parents of children with disabilities because I sometimes forget he is disabled. He approaches life very positively and never gives one the impression he is physically challenged."

A short time later, we found ourselves making preparations to receive our very first international exchange student "daughter," a timid girl from Turkey. Her name was Gokce Gursoy and she was a mere sixteen years old.

When she first arrived, she wasn't sure how she should act around Steven. There was a marked difference between the way she was used to dealing with disabled people in her country versus how we treated Steven. In fact, this was a totally new experience for her. "In my country we don't have a lot of facilities for the disabled, and you don't see them outside their homes very often. My first surprise was that Steve was smoking back then and it was very cold outside, maybe negative twenty degrees Celsius. He had to go outside to smoke. That was the rule in the Hendry house and the rules applied to everybody. He used to stand up really slowly, get dressed, put on his shoes, and go out. This would take him almost twenty minutes. Nobody felt sorry for him or relaxed the rules because he had challenges. He was treated the same as everyone else and was expected to follow the rules. (Smoking is still a habit we are trying to have him break; unfortunately from time to time he turns to cigarettes when his life gets a little too stressful for him.) I was also surprised to find that Steven played a little wheelchair basketball. At that time we did not have such a thing in Turkey. However, we do now. Turkey has come a long way in recent years with respect to access and tolerance for those with disabilities." Gokce was also was surprised at the efforts to make sidewalks, roads, and intersections more accessible to the physically challenged. She quickly learned to adapt, and she and Steven got along famously.

Nikki Wholman (née Krowitz) was our second exchange daughter. She hailed from Johannesburg, South Africa. She was the first of our exchange students to attend Steven's high school, Bluevale Collegiate. Nikki was a very beautiful blonde, blue-eyed girl who turned many heads when she entered a room. Steven told us about the day he was with several of his classmates in the cafeteria during lunch break doing what teenage boys do—clowning around, talking about sports and girls. He recalls how the conversation stopped abruptly when this very attractive "new girl" entered the room. The discussion then turned to "Wow" and "Man, would I like to meet her." Steven gained instant status when he informed this group of awestruck friends, "Yeah, she's pretty cool. Actually I already know her since she lives with us." With

Nikki on the scene, Steven instantly became one of the most popular boys in the school.

Nikki and Steven became very close friends, spending many hours talking about life in high school. Nikki remembers Steven in this way: "I was privileged to spend a year getting to know Steve and living with his family while on Rotary Exchange in 1991. His parents John and Linda were my host parents, and I lived with them a total of six fabulous months. Steve was, and still is, a source of such inspiration to me. He has a love of life that is infectious when you are with him. His tenacity and strength of spirit is also remarkable. Steve never lets anything get him down. When he was working in a job that didn't work out, he went right out and found another one. He never moaned and complained, even when he was required to spend a day on his feet working at the Gap, and this must have been difficult for him. Steve also has a terrific sense of humor, and we spent many hours laughing and joking together. His take on life is truly amazing; he has a positive and lasting impact on all those he meets, and I am so proud to know him."

Another of our exchange students during that period was Sandrine Schneider (née Larrayoz) from France. Sandrine offered her perspective on living with Steven: "Things are not so good for handicapped people in France. Our culture tends to treat persons with disabilities as having a poor quality of life and unable to do many things. This attitude is due in part to the education system in France that doesn't encourage tolerance or provide many accommodations for people with challenges. Steven was very lucky to have a loving family. I noticed they never made special concessions for him and never allowed him to use his disability as an excuse for his behavior or results in school. This environment helped him become autonomous; in their eyes he was a person. I couldn't believe how popular he was in school; it seemed everyone wanted to be his friend. I can't remember a day going by that one of his friends wasn't at the house.

"My most memorable moment with Steven was the time we went to a Guns N' Roses concert in Hamilton, Ontario. I can only imagine what some of the people attending the concert thought of this young

French girl and two other teens, one sitting in a wheelchair, sitting in this crowd of very loud and very scary individuals. Steven was amazing as he sat there cheering, clapping, and singing along with everyone else. The people in the crowd didn't seem to have any influence on him whatsoever. He is very self-confident and reminds me of the adage, 'What doesn't kill you makes you stronger.' He is definitely one of the strongest persons I know."

The year Steven was in grade twelve, a local Japanese tour guide and interpreter, who was also the wife of a prominent photographer and Rotarian, approached Linda and me to see if we might be interested in hosting the daughter of a friend of hers from Japan. The parents were looking for a family in Canada that would take care of their young daughter while she attended summer school and gained experience in a foreign culture. She was only fifteen at the time so it was critical she stay with a trustworthy, caring family that would accept her into their home and look after her like she was their own child.

Linda and I had already planned a trip to Japan that September so we decided we would travel to Kobe to meet Yurika Ogata (née Sawai) and her family. It would give all of us an opportunity to meet each other and get a sense of whether or not a full summer in Canada would work. It also gave her family peace of mind that their daughter was with a good family and would be safe while so far from home. We bonded instantly and it was decided that she would spend the following summer with us.

Yurika's stay with us was a great experience for Steven as he had someone to talk to throughout most of the day; her English skills were excellent. We traveled every weekend to various tourist sites including Toronto and Niagara Falls, and went on multiple shopping excursions. Steven loved the travel because he enjoyed the tourist areas as much as the tourists; it was like each visit was his first. Yurika spent a lot of evenings with the family talking about her experiences, her impressions of Canada, and her home across the world in Kobe. Steven was always ready to partake in a conversation, so the two of them got along famously.

Yurika, living in Tokyo and now married to one of Japan's foremost fashion designers, Yoshiyuki Ogata, reflected on her time living with us, and getting to know Steven: "The summer I lived at the Hendry's I was so impressed that Steven didn't receive any special attention, nor was he treated any different than David or Scott when they were visiting. It seemed to be natural for the family not to give special treatment to the son with a disability. I knew that if I was the one who had a son with a problem walking I think I would always want to help him and ask him if he was okay—even if I knew it would make him feel bad. While I lived with John, Linda, and Steven, I really felt everyone in the family seemed to have a wonderful relationship of love and trust with Steve. He did everything he could manage without expecting anyone to help, and the family offered him assistance only after he asked for it. The family always watched over him with gentle patience—such a great family!"

Megan Brooke, a teen from South Africa was our third Rotary exchange student from Johannesburg. Steven seemed to find satisfaction and a sense of peace by talking to her about what was going on at school. They would spend hours talking about their day at school or activities they were involved in. Although she was a high school student, being from a foreign country she understood the isolation that can be experienced from time to time when you are even slightly different. They shared a keen interest in drama and spent hours discussing the teachers and drama programs at Bluevale. Even after Megan moved to another host family, they kept in close contact with each other throughout her year in Canada. "The thing I remember most about Steven," recalls Megan, "is his smile. To me he was always happy, no matter what his current circumstances seemed to be. He's the kind of person you want to be around just because of the positive energy he gives off. Every time I saw Steve I would feel that infectious smile begin to spread across my face in response to his. I'm sure there must have been times when he was angry or upset and depressed, but as much as I stretch my mind I just can't seem to remember any of those moments. All my memories of Steve are of smiles and laughter and the feeling that he was genuinely grateful to have such a loving family and friends. Steve always expressed an interest in me and my life and made me feel special. He has that way about him—letting you in and blessing you with his Steve-ness."

FRIENDS, BASKETBALL, AND FALLING DOWN STAIRS

Linda and I have hosted students from Japan, Turkey, China, South Africa, Australia, France, Finland, Germany, and Brazil. The students who either stayed with us or that we have met through other exchange students have substantially enriched the lives of everyone in our family. In total twenty-five students have shared our home and become part of our family. Their presence has also had a remarkable impact on Steven's life. Our last student, Nastashia Schoo, from Mount Gambier in the State of South Australia, came to us when Steven was in college, but that didn't deter him from getting to know his new "exchange sister."

Nastashia was a young woman who was politically astute, outspoken, charming, and remarkably popular with her fellow exchange students. She attended Steven's old high school, Bluevale Collegiate, and very soon made countless friends. It didn't take long before she learned that Steven Hendry was legend around the school.

Even though Steven was spending a lot less time at home now, he and Nastashia passed a lot of quality time together, talking for hours about everything from high school to situations in her native Australia and everything in between. Their bond had a great deal to do with the remarkable focus each one of them had. Both were very confident and knew what they wanted, and both were armed with that sense of unstoppable determination. When asked about her memories of Steven she told me, "I remember his bravery and perseverance. It always astonished me, the way he would never back down from pursuing any of his dreams or convictions. His character reminds me of a famous quote by Nelson Mandela: 'I learned that courage was not the absence of fear but the triumph over it.'"

It was our practice at the time to invite our exchange daughters to accompany Steven and me to hockey games. Steven loved all sports and had a keen sense of competition. He was a walking dictionary of both professional and college basketball. His brothers taught him about professional football, which he now follows as avidly as basketball, and he also took an interest in my favorite sport, hockey. I was very involved with the local junior hockey club (the level prior to making the move to professional hockey) and always wanted to expose our students to the excitement of the games. Nastashia was quite eager to join us, at least once, to see if she was interested in the sport or not. She loved the games and became a regular fan with Steven, missing games only once in a while. The hockey game gave her an opportunity to spend a little more time with Steven to carry on their seemingly endless conversations.

Stash, as she's affectionately known by her friends, shared this with me about those Friday night hockey games, "I have this mental image of when we would climb the stairs to our seats. I remember seeing Steven arrive at the auditorium and thinking I should rush down and help him with the steep climb. I quickly learned it was only my perception that needed help. He climbed the stairs with his crutches without batting an eye and found his seat next to me. It seems people with disabilities, in a sense, are more capable of achieving goals because they are so determined. Steven never saw problems; he only saw solutions."

I couldn't have said it better myself.

CHAPTER FIVE

Handling Life's Highs and Lows

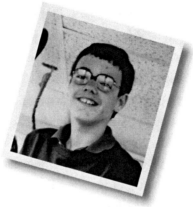

Character cannot be developed in ease and quiet. Only through experience of trial and suffering can the soul be strengthened, vision cleared, ambition inspired, and success achieved.

Helen Keller

We wanted Steven to have strong character. We realized that his life would be a series of ups and downs, and how he faced those ups and downs would determine how he dealt with bigger problems and setbacks later in life. Meeting his struggles and challenges head-on, we explained, would make him a stronger person. It would be easy for him, or for any other person with challenges, to accept help or let others provide assistance rather than making an attempt to overcome a problem himself. If he were to do that, he risked giving up his independence and self-sufficiency. However, accepting help when it is needed makes perfect sense; after all, knowing your limitations is part of self-sufficiency and independence. Fortunately for us, Steven shared our philosophy and practiced it with little influence from us.

MORE, AND MORE, AND MORE SURGERY

The year Steven was eighteen, he underwent another surgery to stabilize his other leg. It was basically the same surgery as the previous one. He had very little muscle tissue in the leg and the weight of his body plus the stress of walking forced the knee to turn, or rotate, inward. This second operation surgically corrected this condition by temporarily installing a metal plate in his knee to stabilize the leg. The hope was that in time his knee would become strong enough to be able to withstand the pressure of walking. Just as with the last one, Dr. Israel coordinated it all and off Steven went to McMaster Medical Center in Ontario.

Like every other surgery preceding this one, he faced it bravely. His disappointment was that he would be missing school and his friends. As we drove to Hamilton, the conversation focused on what was going on at school. We weren't sure if he was simply avoiding talking about the impending operation or had already accepted the time he would be away and was anxious to "get it over with." His attitude left us feeling very proud.

Linda stayed in Hamilton over night the day following the surgery. It was a very long day for both of us. She spent her time in the visitor's lounge waiting to be notified when he was out of surgery; meanwhile I spent my day at work waiting for the phone call from Linda letting me know how the operation went and that Steven he was okay. Finally, after several hours the nursing staff informed Linda that the surgery went well and Steven was in recovery. For Linda his time in recovery seemed to last considerably longer than usual. She was told that he was fine, but they were keeping him in recovery a little longer as a precaution because of the length of time he was in surgery.

In order to keep his mind off the pain, he kept himself occupied planning what he was going to do when he got back to school. He was getting ready to graduate; he was occupied with what he was going to do next in his life. In between flirting with the nurses, he decided to put our theories to good use. He kept his mind focused on remaining positive. During his recovery, he had plenty of time for quiet reflection: "I remembered what mom and dad always told me—what doesn't kill you makes you stronger." There were no idle moments for him; he would set some goals and then devise a strategy to achieve them. When asked about this he commented, "Watching television didn't seem to dull the pain, but thinking about my future plans occupied my mind and forced my pain into the background. Sometimes I would be interrupted by the nurses or the doctor asking if I needed medication for the pain, or to change dressings. I would be okay with the procedure of changing the dressings, but most times I would decline their offer for the pain medication. They would always ask me a second time to make sure I was serious."

Linda and I would stay with him every night in the hospital. Each night we arrived we would hear another story from the nurses. They thought he was hilarious with his constant talking. They were also impressed with his extensive medical knowledge when it came to his procedure. "Does he ever stop talking?" they would ask. They were quite disappointed when the news came that he was to be released to complete his recovery at home.

At home each night there was a steady stream of visitors. Young and old, they would drop in to spend time chatting and catching up. His high school friends would discuss everything from the recent basketball game to the latest gossip in the halls of the school. It was reassuring for Steven to know that he wasn't going to be left out or forgotten. When we look back, it was really quite amazing the way he was accepted and included by his peers.

George Hunsberger, the basketball coach, had grown very close to Steven by this time. He was a constant visitor and turned the tide a bit for Steven during his recovery. Coach Hunsberger wanted to inspire Steven in his recovery as much as Steven had inspired him and his teammates over the years. Their friendship has continued to this day. George recalls, "When Steven's body crumbled past the tolerable level in his grade twelve year, to the extent that once again he had to endure a very painful corrective operation and a long painful recovery period, the basketball team spent many hours wondering what they could do for him. They decided to purchase an official game basketball and have each member sign it. The card said they missed him a lot and that he was still part of the team. The positive effect that this kid had on them as players, and me as coach, and virtually everyone that he came in contact with at the school was truly profound."

For Steven, the feeling was mutual. There was never a day that didn't include some involvement with the basketball team. The team gave him a sense of value and boosted his self-esteem; he believed he was genuinely contributing to something and not just tagging along. There was a valuable lesson for Steven in this; we wanted him to know that the attitude he displayed toward his involvement with the basketball team was the attitude he should have in everything he did. We told him that if he applied that same principle to his everyday living, he would be successful in anything he attempted. "Contribute to the best of your ability and you will always feel that sense of accomplishment," we said. Success can have many faces, and Steven has taught many people the truth of that statement over the years.

LIFELONG FRIENDS AND TRAGEDY

Steven truly was held back by nothing, and while he searched to find the positive in everything, sometimes that wasn't possible in the end. Steven made many friends, but the friends he made as a toddler at the Rotary Centre were some of his closest. Some of these friendships have lasted through into his adulthood. The children attending the center shared a common bond with their exceptionalities, so it was easy for them to become friends. They naturally bonded because of their exceptionalities. They could be themselves, accepting each other for who they were. Two in particular I've mentioned before, Brandy and Jeff. They were Steven's best friends. They spent a great deal of time with each other, like the three musketeers. Amazingly, all three had the same attitude about life and their disabilities. It was the hand they had been dealt and it wasn't going to stop them or even slow them down.

Jeff was a very good-looking young boy with an engaging personality. He was born with spina bifida and although confined to a wheelchair, it didn't stop him from being quite popular at school, particularly with the girls. He was truly an extrovert and always in the thick of things at his school. His mannerisms and attitude were very similar to Steven's and he mingled throughout the entire school population making friends and getting involved. I remember observing him at the shopping mall on weekends where he spent a lot of time with his friends, charming the ladies.

Brandy too was born with cerebral palsy, and like Jeff, she was confined to a wheelchair. But the moment you met her, you knew she was a very intelligent and determined young woman—nothing was going to stand in her way of having a successful life. She was confident and very independent despite her physical challenges. An attractive and articulate young lady, Brandy could hold her own in any debate or discussion. She was also a serious student and focused on academic success.

Tragedy struck just before Christmas, 1993. Jeff had had several operations over the years as a result of his spina bifida. Surgery can be a risk at any time for any person; there are so many things that can go wrong. Jeff always confided in Steven and Brandy that he was terrified and apprehensive about the surgeries. He knew the operations were necessary and each time he bravely accepted the risk. Sadly this surgery proved to be too much for Jeff's fragile body, and he never recovered. It was very difficult for his family and friends to deal with as he was such a big part of their lives, and it was a terrible shock to us all. Jeff's close circle of friends was devastated; they couldn't imagine a world without their buddy.

Steven had a hard time dealing with Jeff's death. When he received the news he couldn't believe it. "How could this happen?" he kept asking. He had never been faced with this kind of tragedy before. It was surreal; perhaps a dream that he would wake up from and find it never happened. It was difficult for him to hide his feelings, one minute they were laughing and having fun, the next Jeff was gone. He didn't talk much about it, which was very unusual for Steven. It was how we knew how hard he was taking his loss. We could see the impact it had on him. He lost his spark a little. In later conversations when he was ready to talk, he told us how he thought about his own mortality. We asked him if he was worried about surgery in the future. He said he wasn't worried, or even upset anymore, he just missed his friend Jeff and it would take a long time to get used to him not hanging out together.

Following Jeff's death, Steven and Brandy really leaned on each other. Brandy thought the world of Steven: "He was a selfless friend in the true sense of the word. Despite dealing with his own demons, he always had time to listen to a friend in need of someone to talk to. There were times that I know Steven really struggled to rebuild and regain his sense of 'self' as we all have. There were times during my highs and lows as a teen, and in early adulthood, where I struggled, trying to make sense of things while driving through such turmoil in my own home life. I remember days and nights when Steven would set aside his tasks and his own concerns for a conversation, a few jokes, or to provide a listening ear or a hug. He was always this constant—and I think there were times when I really put his heart and mind through their paces."

Time as they say always heals, and that was true for Steven as well. As time wore on, he still missed his friend, but his natural verve for life returned. He was able to live life fully, no matter what it threw at him.

"SORRY, THE JOB HAS ALREADY BEEN FILLED"

The older he got, it seemed the more he had to deal with though. While the government has made tremendous advances in accessibility for persons with disabilities; unfortunately tolerance and sensitivity cannot be legislated. Discrimination and bias against individuals with challenges is very much alive in our society. Most times, it is the worst kind of discrimination, the kind that is subtle and cruel. I have since realized that the subtle kind is really nothing more than blatant discrimination dressed up in a well-intentioned lie. I wish I had a dollar for every time I heard the well-meaning comment, "It's great to see someone like him doing so well."

Steven dealt with his fair share of discrimination, both subtle and overt. While I never tried to shield him from it, I also never kept him out of harm's way. Linda and I decided early on that Steven would have to learn to deal with the inevitable. There would be people who would judge him based on his physical condition, no matter how hard he worked or how upbeat he was.

The older he got, the more he was faced with this kind of subtle discrimination. It especially reared its ugly head when it came time for Steven to find a part-time job. He was old enough and definitely capable enough. His friends were all getting jobs, why not him? Like his friends, he had been looking for some time without much success either the type of work was too difficult for him, or the location wasn't convenient for him to get there easily. Eventually, a job at a local pizza restaurant was advertised in the newspaper. Steven felt he could handle the duties and the location was within walking distance, so he decided to apply. The advertisement invited interested individuals to apply by telephone. He made the call and did everything right; he was polite, spoke with a clear, confident voice, and was available at all the key times required for the position. The interviewer told him he had the qualifications and that they liked his attitude and friendly manner. When he inquired about the possibility of a second interview, he was told it wasn't necessary; he was definitely the best candidate, and the job was his if he wanted it. Steven was so excited he volunteered to start within the hour. I drove him over to the restaurant and listened to him describe in detail all the places he was going to spend his money. I was proud of him and very happy to see him so enthusiastic.

Before he got out of the car to go into the restaurant, I gave him some fatherly advice on how to conduct himself and cautioned him to listen very closely to the manager when he gave instructions. Most important, I told him if he wasn't sure or didn't completely understand instructions or duties, to ask. With that, he got out of the car and walked into the restaurant. I waited briefly to make sure he got inside okay and proceeded to back out of the parking spot. The next thing I saw was Steven coming back out into the parking lot. When he opened the car door my first question was, "What did you forget?"

He was noticeably upset, something highly unusual.

"As soon as saw me, the manager made an apology and said it was his assistant manager that had hired me, and he didn't realize the position had already been filled," Steven told me.

> Every individual can advocate for accessibility in the work place. One of the easiest accommodations that can be made is insuring there are sufficient parking spaces for the disabled. When a new facility is being planned, it is the ideal time to include accessibility in the plans. Simple features like lower light switches and door handles can be part of the design and not add any additional cost to the project. Many jurisdictions are now passing laws to insure all new buildings are accessible. This means insuring all entrance doors, emergency exits, and washroom doors permit easy access for wheelchairs. Washrooms also must include lower sinks. When modifications or renovations are being discussed at any public place, including a workspace, don't be afraid to ask the all important question: "Will the change make the business more accessible?" If the parking lot is to be upgraded or expanded insist the curbs be cut to enable wheelchair access. If the building is on a grade, instead of installing a set of steps, add a ramp.
>
> Employers can take the first step to make their business accessible by creating and enforcing an equity and inclusion policy. Acknowledging persons with challenges can fill many roles in an organization, and hiring practices should be based on ability not disability. Employees can help by speaking up when they witness unfair treatment or comments and supporting policies that guarantee inclusion and equity for everyone.

We decided not to jump to conclusions, so we gave them the benefit of the doubt; it certainly could have happened that way. A week later when we received the newspaper, Steven again began to review the help-wanted listings. To our dismay we found the same pizza restaurant ad. There could be no denying it; the manager made an assumption as soon as he saw Steven in person, that Steven wouldn't be able to perform the job. The decision was made without asking Steven or giving him the chance to prove he could perform all the responsibilities and duties of the job. I wanted to make his unfair treatment public knowledge, but Steven refused. He just wanted to move on and look for another job.

Some employers in businesses and industries continue to discriminate against persons with disabilities. The argument in Canada and the United States is that we are ahead of most other countries in the world when it comes to equity, but discrimination too often goes hand in hand with that complacency. Notions of equity can be of little solace to the individual who has been bypassed as a result of ignorance and intolerance, especially in situations where they may have been the most qualified applicant. Many companies avoid being criticized or accused of discriminatory practices by accepting applications and interviewing candidates with disabilities. But if these candidates are not hired, the interviews may be merely smoke screens for acts of discrimination.

We have come a long way, and improvements have been made as demonstrated by the number of persons with disabilities in the workplace today. However, we have a long way to go. It is actually quite a sad commentary on our society to think that we require legislation in order to create a level playing field for candidates who have disabilities.

FINDING HUMOR IN "HANDY"

Steven was disappointed with the manager's behavior, but eventually his good humor got the better of him. Steven's cousin Heather McNab summed up nicely how Steven was able to handle so many adverse situations: "I have a million stories that I could tell but the first word about Steven that always comes to mind is attitude. Regardless what has happened, or is happening to him, he is in a great mood and has a wonderful attitude towards life. No matter how many times he falls, or how much physical or emotional pain he is feeling, he is always willing to talk about it. He doesn't care that people will laugh; in fact he likes it when they do. I believe he is so willing to share his stories because he knows we will all get a big laugh out of them, even if it is at his expense. I still love getting phone calls from him that start with, 'Heady, did I pull a Handy.' I know at that moment I will be laughing hysterically, and Steven will be laughing right along with me."

Steven has referred to himself as "Handyman" (his short form for handicapped man) ever since a mischievous friend presented him with a broken handicapped parking sign as a joke. He doesn't get hung up on political correctness because he feels good about himself. Heather in fact witnessed many of his "Handy" moments as she had traveled with us a couple of times on our yearly pilgrimage to Florida. Many times Steven seemed to become the entertainment for the group with his impromptu antics. Most of the time he accepts the jokes and one-liners as a form of endearment or acceptance.

Heather's mother Maureen, for example, has teased Steven mercilessly throughout his life. She has always paid close attention to him, loving him by poking fun at him, teasing, or just laughing at some of his mannerisms. Steven remains close to Maureen today, and even as an adult, her unrelenting teasing continues. He loves it! He is the first to laugh at himself. Perhaps it started as a form of self-defense. Perhaps, he just came that way and hasn't thought anything about it. But it is undeniable; he has found such pleasure over the years bringing laughter into people's lives that it's become an essential part of who he is. However, don't ever think for a moment this does not in any way suggest that he is not hurt or bothered by insensitive actions or comments. Fortunately for him—and for us—in his wisdom, he knows the difference.

TRAVELING WITH STEVEN

In any physically challenged person's life, they need to learn to adapt. Unfortunately, the rest of the world is still catching up to their uniqueness. I've been told by many parents of challenged children that they have to gently guide their children—and sometime push them kicking and screaming—to experience life outside of their safe zone. Steven was adventurous enough that we never had to prod. Rather, we often had to restrain ourselves. Our annual vacation to Florida was a case in point.

We started going to Florida when Steven was eleven. The drudgery of winter certainly was only one of many motivating factors. We had never been on a family vacation that took us far away from home; Linda had never traveled outside of Canada. Most of our friends had made the trip, some more than once. We finally decided at Christmas that when the annual school spring break rolled around in March of 1983 that we were finally going to make the trip—by car. With two boys and two adults traveling, flying simply wasn't an option.

It seemed that everyone we knew who had made the trip to Florida was prepared to give us advice. Where to stop on the long drive, where not to stop, how to dress, and what potential problems we should be prepared for along the way. One piece of advice that we received from many of our experienced snow-bird friends was "Don't worry about booking motels on the drive down and back. There are plenty of hotels and they are never full." So like any other novice traveler, we accepted their advice and scratched "book motel rooms" from our extensive to-do list.

Finally March rolled around, and the time had come for the Hendry's to strike out on our first family vacation adventure. Unfortunately we didn't have our full family. David, then sixteen, was unable to get time off from his new part-time job working at the local White Rose Nursery. Since it was a new job and he wanted to start saving money, he decided it wouldn't be the best career move to ask for time off. David was very mature and despite our recommendation to stay with his aunt and uncle for the week, he opted to stay at home and fend for himself. We were disappointed he wasn't able to be with us but we also understood how he felt about his job. We knew this might be the last time we could vacation together as a family since the boys would not want to travel with their parents once they reached their mid-teens. But he was resolute, so off we went. Steven was disappointed, but secretly I think he and Scott were also glad—one less body to share the back seat with.

When we look back to that first trip, we realize how we must have appeared to our neighbors. We packed for every seasonal weather condition and disaster imaginable. The trunk was packed to the point that we had to force it shut. When we ran out of room in the trunk, we filled every available space in the back seat not occupied by Scott and Steven. We packed blankets just in case we had car trouble and got stranded. We had plenty of books and games for the boys, and we even packed winter coats and boots (you know, just in case it snowed in Florida in March.)

On a map, driving to Florida is pretty straightforward; simply drive Ontario Highway 401 west to the Windsor/Detroit border, and get on to US Highway I75 and head south through six states to Florida.

We had no idea what to expect as we left the house at three-thirty in the morning. Our hope was to arrive at our destination in approximately twenty-eight to thirty hours with Linda and me sharing the driving. During the trip we stopped every couple hours for stretching and fuel; while one drove, the other used the time to sleep. The boys didn't seem to mind the discomfort of riding in the back seat of the car, falling asleep quite easily.

As daylight broke on our first full day on the road, we were driving through the mountains of Tennessee. The scenery was breathtaking. Steven and Scott, much to our surprise, were behaving themselves in their cramped quarters. It was surprising to us that the two boys were not having any territorial disputes, at least not yet. Both boys passed the time reading books, listening to their favorite music, or sleeping.

Finally the long trip began to take a toll on Linda and me. Changing drivers frequently was helping, but we weren't really able to sleep comfortably in the car. The reality that we would not be able to drive straight through to Florida was finally becoming a fact. Of course, according to our friends, finding a motel would not be a problem. By the time we accepted the fact that we could not safely carry on, we had arrived in northern Florida, but motel after motel displayed the depressing sign, "No Vacancies."

Shortly after midnight, one full day after we left home, we arrived in Gainesville, Florida. We were totally exhausted and still could not find a room. We found out there was a university festival being held in the Gainesville area and every motel was full. In desperation we pulled into the parking lot of a Holiday Inn and spent the night sleeping in the car. The boys, ever resilient, thought it was pretty cool. It was one of the most uncomfortable nights Linda and I had ever spent, and it was rapidly taking the excitement out of our first Florida trip.

The next morning we walked across the parking lot to a restaurant for breakfast, and after a quick bite we were back on the road. Finally, some four hours later we arrived at our destination on Anna Maria Island. The boys were excited; Linda and I were relieved. In the backs of our minds we were thinking, "Six days from now we are going to be facing that long drive again!"

In the many trips south in subsequent years, we stayed at motels for at least two nights to give Steven (and his mother and father) a bit of a break.

At this point in his life, Steven used both the wheelchair and his forearm crutches. The wheelchair was used when he was required to cover longer distances or for extended periods of time too long for him to be on his feet. During these lengthy trips to Florida, he used his crutches while exercising his legs at rest stops and to get to and from the car. Packing the car always required a little patience and creativity as we also had to make sure that whatever luggage we took with us, there was still room for Steven's wheelchair in the trunk of the car.

Each stop we made Steven would walk with his crutches and try to work the stiffness out of his legs, hips, and back. He never complained about the pain or discomfort we were sure he was feeling. This was an adventure for him and he was excited. Stopping at restaurants was always a time for Steven to turn on the charm with the waitresses. He loved to talk, and they intently listened. It didn't really matter what the subject was, Steven would somehow find a way to carry on a lengthy conversation. We were assured the level of service was always going to be top notch when he traveled with us.

Linda and I were always proud of the way he conducted himself. He was courteous and polite, almost to a fault, thanking people when they held doors open for him or tried to help him get to his feet on those occasions where he lost his balance and took a tumble. Naturally, people would want to help him regain his footing, but he would politely say "No, thank you. I'm okay." It was part of his "I'm normal" attitude and confidence. Normal people didn't need help getting up when they fell, so by extension he didn't either. Incidentally, he fell a lot! There were a multitude of causes for his falling including uneven pavement, stepping on a stone or rock, or being bumped. However, the most common reason for his spills was his own inattention—he was so into what was going on around him that he occasionally lost his balance or trip over something. We never scolded him for it—how could we? That would have broken his spirit and that was never part of the game plan. If he had bumps and bruises, so what? Bodies heal, even ones with cerebral palsy.

WHAT MEDICAL CONDITION?

We regularly stayed in a condominium resort called Runaway Bay on a pretty little island south of Tampa, on the Gulf of Mexico. The resort had many amenities including shuffle board and a swimming pool. Steven loved playing shuffle board. I think it was because he could use the paddle as a crutch to steady himself; he liked to try walking without crutches from time to time. (His gait when he walked without his crutches was most peculiar indeed; it always drew somewhat guarded looks from others around him.) Although a little shaky, he managed to play the game without assistance, just like everyone else. Every now and then we would make special allowances like letting him have a second shot to get closer to the end of the board. Usually making special concessions were a no-no, but we all figured we were on vacation, it was the best time to relax the rules a bit. He loved being able to participate with everyone else playing whether they were children or adults.

The one place he really thrived was in the water where he would enjoy freedom with little discomfort. He would spend hours in the pool emerging with fingers and toes wrinkled like prunes only after we insisted or if it was time to eat. (As much as Steven loved the water, he also loved to eat.) In the water he was in his element, and it made him very happy. I'm sure there were many times when the other visitors in the complex must have thought we abandoned him, given how long he stayed in the pool.

The evenings were spent going for walks in the warm Gulf breeze, enjoying the white sand, the sound of the surf, watching the people, and poking through the shops that dotted the island. One particular night, the resort was holding their regular weekly bingo night. I was never a bingo fan but Steven, always the inquisitive type, had to investigate. The first thing he noticed was that he was well below the average age of most of the people in the room. There were perhaps two other children but it was apparent they were not there of their own free will.

Not one to let shyness get the better of him, Steven took up a position next to the bingo's organizer, intently watching as he spun the numbered balls in the barrel and then drew one out. "Can I help you?"

This was an unusual question coming from Steven since most often it was someone asking that of him. His charm and personality were always disarming so the next thing we knew, he was spinning the barrel and reaching in to pull out the balls. However, the organizer drew the line at Steven's request that he call out the numbers too. On some of those evenings, he would spend hours participating in the bingo games and chatting with the players, most of them old enough to be his grandparents.

Driving to Florida the year Steven was fifteen, he was uncharacteristically quiet. At first we weren't too concerned and took advantage of the peace and quiet to discuss other things going on at the time. However, he virtually stopped eating, complaining he wasn't hungry. As we drew closer to Florida, his condition seemed to worsen. His temperature continued to increase, and he stopped talking altogether choosing instead to sleep. The telltale red spots and fever soon gave it away: Steven had contracted chicken pox. Fortunately, we'd already had them, but Steven was going to be contagious to others at the resort, so once we'd arrived, he was forced to stay indoors until the worst of it was over. We felt badly for him because these trips to Florida were a time for him to let loose a bit and enjoy his time away from the rigor of therapy and school. The weather was perfect that week with sunshine every day and temperatures in the high eighties. We had difficulty enjoying ourselves because in the back of our minds we couldn't stop thinking of Steven stuck in the condo.

But instead of complaining, he found something to be interested in to occupy his time—basketball. He was still a freshman in high school when this all happened, and this is when he learned to love the sport that would give so much back to him over the years. The first afternoon he spent on his own, he discovered the art of channel-surfing on the television. It didn't take very long for him to find the sports channel. This happened to be the biggest week of the year in the United States for college basketball. The NCAA (National College Athletic Association) Sweet Sixteen tournament was televised throughout the entire week. Steven was very adept in picking up the nuances of almost every sport, so by the end of the week he knew every competing team, their hometown, and their national ranking. He would report on the score of every game, and could name every team's key players. It was truly amazing the way he absorbed so much information on one sport in such a short period of time. From that day forward, he could become involved in conversations with anyone familiar with the game of basketball or the NCAA championship tournament.

By our second week there, Steven was no longer contagious—freedom at last! Unfortunately, the weather had taken a turn for the worse. For the first time in the several years we'd been going to Florida, we were forced to endure several days of cool rainy weather that kept everyone out of the Gulf, as well as the swimming pool. Our activities for the rest of the week were restricted to the indoors. It wasn't what any of us, particularly Steven, had in mind for a Florida vacation. As depressing as the situation was, Steven didn't complain. Instead, he was convinced he was going to be able to go on some kind of fast-forward program in order to catch up on the activities he had missed.

There are times when one's principles are tested. For example, Linda and I have always suggested that we trusted Steven to do the right thing, to make decisions that were well thought out, and to never take unnecessary chances when it came to trying new things. That guidance always seemed to work when it applied to Steven's choices. However, it was thoroughly tested the year he was fifteen. Steven was constantly exploring new experiences, and it seemed to me at the time that these adventures were always of the dangerous variety. We were about to get our first taste of this quest for adventure.

Although we traveled to Florida every year we only took in the theme parks every second or third year. On those occasions we would take in Disney World, Universal Studios, or Busch Gardens. Linda and I felt so bad for Steven being shut-in the previous week, so we decided to break that routine and take the boys to Disney World. It couldn't replace the week he had just lost, but it would certainly take the edge off it.

It was a three hour trip from the Sarasota area to Orlando, meaning we had to get up very early and be on our way if we were going to get full value for our day at Disney World. Steven was not a morning person and as anxious as he was to "be there," he wasn't terribly excited about being awakened at five o'clock in the morning. However as we drove his mood gradually returned to normal. This meant talking as long as someone was listening.

On the drive, he casually advised us he couldn't wait to ride Space Mountain at Disney World, a ride definitely not for the faint of heart.

We wondered if he told the whole truth when queried by the attendant whose job it was to check and make sure that people entering the ride met the health and safety criteria. The attendant would ask, "Do you have any medical conditions that would cause discomfort or worse? Do you have any back injuries that might possibly be aggravated by this ride?" Steven confidently assured them that he was fine and would not be in any danger. The fact that he was riding in a wheelchair and then transferring to crutches never appeared to raise any red flags with the attendants. I could never understand what it was that tipped the scale for him to be allowed on the ride. I was always hoping they would politely turn him away while deep in my heart I remember how proud I was of him for his courage and tenacity. He always seemed to be able to convince them, and me, that he wouldn't be in any imminent danger and that he had been on similar rides many times without incident. Space Mountain was one of the top attractions at the theme park and truly an adventure. It was two-and-a-half minutes of lightning speed, hairpin turns, and sudden drops in altitude that threw the rider back against the seat with tremendous force.

If you've ever been to Disney World, you know Space Mountain The ride posed some risk even for healthy riders. However, for a youngster with physical challenges, and riding in a wheelchair, the risk factor increased dramatically. We imagined a multitude of things that could go wrong or sudden movements that he couldn't possibly prepare for, each one of them capable of inflicting serious harm to him. Reluctantly, I consented with the caveat that the final decision would be made by Linda—after all, mothers know best! She had a lot more faith in his judgment and bravado than I, and of course, most of the time she was right.

So off he went with his brother Scott to conquer Space Mountain. I remember silently hoping the long wait in line would dampen his enthusiasm, and he would change his mind, or that when he arrived at the entrance, the attendant would turn him away out of fear of his being injured. That didn't happen.

In what seemed like an eternity, the two prevailing heroes emerged from the base of the mountain with smiles stretching from ear to ear. Scott told us it went really well after he helped Steven and the attendant place Steven securely into the seat. He then told us about how excited and loud Steven was as they catapulted along the dark path of the ride. They both loved it, and we were convinced that the ride signaled a major bonding experience for them both. The two of them would brave the ride at least twice more on that day. No matter how many times we visited the park, they never got tired of it; in fact, if we weren't insistent, they would take the ride until the park closed. Whether he was with his brother, a friend, or an exchange student, no matter who joined him, he always exited the mountain sporting an enormous grin and begging us to allow him to go one more time.

For Steven, there was never a question of whether or not he would be safe. He clearly realized his limitations and reassured me each time, saying, "I'll be okay, Dad. Don't worry." And away he would go, disappearing into the line.

Disney World is filled with thrilling rides like Space Mountain and Steven made it his goal to try every single one of them. Life is of course filled with many little adventures. For some, Disney World would only signify a fun family vacation. For me, the times we spent at the Magic Kingdom became a turning point. I truly believe it had a profound influence on Steven's attitude toward life. Not only did he accomplish something daring. On the rides he was no different than the person sitting next to him. He had nothing to prove. I don't know if he even thought about that. His only thought was to have fun and move on to the next ride, but it meant the world to me. I have always found it was fitting that Space Mountain was situated in "Tomorrowland," fitting because Steven strongly believed his life would be different tomorrow and that everything going on around him at the time was magic.

Watching Steven handle all that he had to—the constant physical pain, the torment of subtle discrimination, the loss of his dear friend, a loss we all have to suffer at some point in our lives—I realized that to me, Steven embodied one of my favorite quotes, by Meg Cabot:

Courage is not the absence of fear but the judgment that something else is more important than fear. The brave may not live forever but the cautious do not live at all. For now you are traveling the road between who you think you are and who you can be.

I learned a lot about courage from Steven, and by watching him, by standing aside most of the time, by stepping in when necessary, I have learned more about who I am as well. What better gift can a son give a father?

CHAPTER SIX
Closing in on the Destination

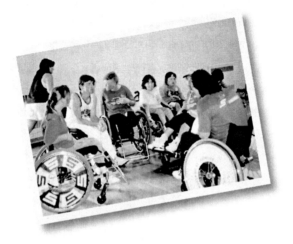

All of life is a journey which paths we take, what we look back on, and what we look forward to is up to us. We determine our destination, and what kind of road we will take to get there, and how happy we are when we get there.

Author Unknown

As Steven's high school years were coming to a close, he was busy making plans, like all high-school seniors do, for college. Most colleges and universities in the United States and Canada have a program whereby students with physical or intellectual challenges can apply for entry. The application and acceptance process is modified to consider the applicants' academic standing in the context of their challenges while still preserving the minimum standards of the college.

Steven had planned to attend college for a long time, in part because his high school friends would be moving on to either college or university. However, he also had more realistic goals, such as preparing himself for a future career. He realized with his disabilities, it was going to be very difficult to find meaningful employment if all he had to offer was a high school diploma. The opportunities available to him would definitely improve if could add a college diploma to his résumé.

Grade twelve proved to be a little more difficult than Steven had expected, yet another setback. While some of his marks were good, unfortunately, others were not so good and dragged his average down slightly below the benchmark for college acceptance. Naturally, he was disappointed and decided to talk to the guidance counselor at the high school. At about this time, Conestoga College in Kitchener, Ontario, contacted him and informed him that even though his marks were low, he would be able to enter the college by applying through their Disability Entrance Program.

We expected he would be overjoyed at the news, but he wasn't. He felt he had the ability to do much better, and if he had to enter the college any other way but through the "front door," he wouldn't do it. Instead, following his meeting with the counselor, he decided to return to Bluevale Collegiate for one more semester to improve his marks so that he could apply to the college the same as every one of his friends had to. His pride and self-assurance would not allow him to take the easy route—he wanted to earn his place at the college. While he felt the Disability Entrance Program was a terrific opportunity for students who otherwise would have difficulty qualifying as a result of the degree of their challenge, in his heart he knew he had the ability to qualify for acceptance the same as most other students. He just had to apply himself and earn it!

Since he had a specific goal in mind, he was able to work hard focus on his math and English to improve his marks. In order to accomplish this goal, it meant he had to be willing to sacrifice. That meant asking for help and remaining after school or going in early. Our suggestion was to ask a question when he didn't understand something in class. I remember telling him as he struggled with his math homework, "It's like building a house; you start from the ground up—one level at a time! Take the time to understand each step of a problem, then soon it will seem like someone just turned on a light and you will understand and be ready to move on to the next level."

He applied the same principle to his English class. Steven had the good fortune of having teachers that were willing to give him the extra help and extra time he required to understand the course material. The secret of course was really quite simple and could be summed up in one

> Most colleges and universities today have policies regarding the provision of equal access for all students despite their disabilities. Their services insure that a student's needs are met including the provision of adaptive technology, FM systems, note takers, tutors, test proctors, test accommodations or modifications, alternative print formats, and a variety of software to help those with learning disabilities. They also make sure the students' special requirements are well documented and communicated to the faculty. Conestoga College, by last count, has a list of forty-one accommodations available to assist students with special needs.
>
> In the past, many students with disabilities have been prevented from attending college or university because the buildings or location were not accessible. Today most provinces and states in Canada and the US have passed laws forcing publicly funded facilities to be accessible for everyone. As the parent of a child with physical challenges, I would be the first to suggest it is impossible to make all facilities accessible. At times governments also have to consider what is reasonable when considering modifying existing facilities.
>
> The student also has a responsibility to make his or her needs known, and to report issues that are barriers to their learning environment.

word—ask! We know it was difficult for him because it meant overcoming his friends' requests to go out to the movies or hang out. Whenever he felt tempted to skip a night he reminded himself of his goal as well as the pay-off, acceptance to college. We were quite impressed with his dedication and commitment, and grateful to the teachers. He finished he extra year at Bluevale Collegiate, and his grades were good enough. He was going to college on his own merit.

A TOUGH RIDE

Probably, in the back of his mind, Steven thought college would be an extension of his high school experience, with few changes in his social life or extracurricular involvement. Unfortunately his expectations were a little oversimplified, and it didn't take long to find it was going to be a lot more difficult than he had anticipated. According to Steven, "I figured as long as I enjoyed learning about business, I would find the classes and assignments easy, or at least manageable. It wasn't that way at all. I faced challenges I hadn't experienced in a long time such as mathematics. I thought I had mastered the concepts of math after struggling with it for a long time in high school, but here it was again. It took at lot of frustrating sessions with the teacher and a lot of work at home to understand the concepts at the college level. At times I felt like quitting, like I would never get it. I began to doubt myself and wondered if I had maybe bit off more than I could chew. However, with the help of the teachers, a few of my classmates, and the constant encouragement from my mom and dad, I worked my way through it."

The problems Steven was experiencing in college were really not unlike those faced by his peers. Students at some point in their college or university career discover an area that becomes a challenge for them. We tried to encourage Steven to just take it one step at a time and continue asking for help from either his teachers or another student when he needed it. But most important, we urged him to make every effort to find a solution to the problem himself. It was a concept he had embraced throughout his life to this point, and it had served him well in this situation too.

At first, college life was a letdown for Steven. This was a surprise for all of us. Steven told me, "Even though I had lots of friends, I felt isolated while at school. There wasn't a lot of opportunity for me to be social. Unlike high school where there was always a strong sense of belonging, I found it very difficult to fit in at college. There were so many students from so many social circles."

Like his father, Steven loved to be involved, to express his opinions, and bring about change. It didn't take long for Steven to find a place where he could belong and even make a difference. As a result of his extroverted personality, Steven was asked if he would like to become a student representative on the College Special Needs Advisory Committee, a position he eagerly accepted. "I had strong opinions about issues that students with disabilities faced and often took a stand not readily accepted by the college. I learned a life lesson quickly. Bringing about change is not easy; it takes hard work, patience, and respect for others' opinions, and compromise if you want to effect change or solve problems."

The course of study Steven selected was Business Co-op. His goal was to work in an office environment after graduation and hopefully move into a management position with a progressive company. His plans never took "disabilities" or "challenges" into consideration since he felt he could compete for a job, or function in any management position that another individual might.

His first placement in the co-op program was at the college in the Liaison and Information Services Department. He thoroughly enjoyed the experience. "I played an important role in planning an orientation weekend for incoming first-year students. I loved it! My task was to plan an event that would give new students a good first impression of the college. It was quite a responsibility; the work was hard but I excelled at it. I was convinced business and working with people were my strengths. The best lesson I learned from it was the importance of taking responsibility for your work ethic and effort and taking pride in your accomplishments," Steven expressed.

One of the most difficult challenges Steven had in college was how to not get too stressed out. Stress comes from being overwhelmed by too many tasks at hand. Steven was never a very well organized person. Like many people with learning disabilities, he was constantly challenged by his lack of organizational skills. Unfortunately, he could only manage to take on one task at a time. Attempting to simultaneously complete a number of tasks would almost always have disastrous results. At times, when we sensed he was feeling a little overwhelmed, we would suggest he "take a step back" and refocus, completing one task at a time. Linda would always tell Steven, "Take a deep breath, start with the task you have to complete first and work on it until it is finished, then move on to the next one." Once he started forcing himself to organize in that manner, his stress level was reduced substantially.

The post-secondary experience wasn't all bad for Steven; there were more positives than negatives along the way. "College itself, despite the challenges I faced, taught me a lot about working hard if I wanted to be successful. It taught me to understand what my limits were, to do the very best I could to expand those limits, and to finally accept them and move ahead with my life. Attending college was a critical time in life for me because it allowed me the opportunity to see for myself what my own challenges were, and with that knowledge create a way to find success."

DRIVING—A "LIFE-ALTERING" EXPERIENCE

Steven had to depend on his friends, family, and public transportation to get around but he didn't like to impose on anyone. He always felt guilty asking for rides, so if he had any money he would take a cab, not wanting to inconvenience us. He would always say that we had done enough for him and that the least he could do was take public transportation. One day out of the blue, he suggested to us that he had decided he would like to learn to drive. We were not as surprised as one might expect; after all this was a boy who defied the odds throughout his life. However, this time we knew he was going to face insurmountable roadblocks, not the least of which was the fact that he was quadriplegic.

In order to get a learner's permit, persons with physical challenges must pass a reflex test. The test was a series of physical movements performed by a medical technician at the hospital. The purpose is to determine if an individual with mobility problems has the ability to safely operate a vehicle in stressful situations such as applying the brakes or steering to avoid a collision. For Steven the issue was going to be moving his leg from the gas pedal to the brake pedal quickly enough to pass. He required significant effort to move his leg successfully. Fortunately for him he was able to pivot his foot quite easily on his heel in order to transfer from the gas to the break. He understood the risk of disappointment if he failed the test, but he also said if he didn't try he would never know, so he made the appointment. Several weeks later he had his reflex test. Waiting for the results proved to be more stressful for him than the actual test. Not to our surprise, he remained cautiously optimistic; in fact he was sure he would pass.

Linda and I talked about it; we were both sure Steven would not get past this particular challenge. He was quadriplegic and had limited use of his legs. How could he possibly get over this hurdle?

Much to our surprise, he passed the reflex test, meeting the standard for physically challenged drivers. The only accommodation he required was a "spinner." Spinners, popular with the "cool" drivers back in the fifties, allow the driver to turn corners easily by not having to take his or her hands off the steering wheel at any time. They have since been banned and can only be used by a physically challenged driver with a special permit.

Steven checked the phone book for driving schools that offered programs to the physically challenged. He managed to find one that on the surface appeared to be a competent school with experienced professional instructors. It was, however, a disaster and a major setback for Steven's self-confidence. The driving instructor was definitely not cut out to teach persons with special needs. In fact, after listening to some of the stories Steven told relating to his lessons, I doubt this particular instructor was cut out to teach anyone to drive. He definitely had communication issues and was very nervous driving with Steven (that part I understood). The company seemed to have little problem accepting his money but had major problems providing meaningful instruction. It was becoming very depressing for Steven, and he became more and more frustrated with every passing day. For whatever reason the instructor was just not able to provide instructions that he understood, and the costs were beginning to add up.

True to his personality, he refused to give up. Nothing was going to prevent him from learning to drive. He would worry about passing the driving test later. After weeks of frustration, he reluctantly decided the

CLOSING IN ON THE DESTINATION

driving school was not going to work. He made it clear he wasn't giving up; it just wasn't going to happen at this particular driving school.

It never once crossed my mind that he would ask me to teach him to drive. His choice was based on his mother's advice (I could never thank her enough for her confidence), and economics; he had used all the money he had on the last driving school and didn't want to risk spending more money trying to find a school that could help him. Many years before, early in our marriage, I had worked part-time as a driving instructor with a fairly impressive success rate. I had never instructed anyone with physical challenges, though, and had never been brave enough to teach anyone without the safety feature of a set of dual breaks.

I knew Steven's persistence and determination would eventually wear me down, so I gave in and agreed to at least try. Little did I know it was to become a life-altering experience. Unlike Steven's previous instructor, I started him in the parking lot of the local arena just to be sure we completely understood each other and that he was totally familiar with the vehicle. The critical key in teaching Steven to drive was going to be awareness or "defensive driving." I made the assumption before he got behind the wheel of the car that his reaction times were going to be significantly slower than other new drivers. It was imperative that Steven consciously allowed extra time for sudden changes in conditions.

As a driving instructor, you learn very quickly never to assume your student understands your explicit instructions. Situations occur instantaneously and you always had to be ready to make rapid corrections. We agreed that there would be key commands that Steven would carry out immediately without question. This rule was intended to assure our survival as well as the survival of other drivers on the road. My life passed before my eyes on many occasions, but I never lost my temper or shouted at him. I was so impressed with his desire to learn and his unyielding determination that I figured I owed him every possible chance to achieve this lofty goal. We had a few close calls, numerous brushes with the curb, and a few near misses.

On one occasion I asked Steven to make a left turn from a four-lane road onto a quieter street. He checked for traffic behind him, looked over his shoulder checking his blind spot, and proceeded to change lanes. He made only one mistake; the lane he so perfectly moved into was actually the passing lane for oncoming traffic. I grabbed the steering wheel and abruptly moved to the right avoiding a potentially serious accident. I remained calm, but I could feel my heart pounding in my chest. I noticed Steven's hands were shaking from the near collision and he apologized for the next several minutes. I assured him the mistake he just made is made by many people every day. The important outcome was to remember why it happened and make sure to not make the same mistake in the future.

One snowy Sunday afternoon, we had just started his lesson when we decided to take on some driving conditions that were a little more challenging. We headed for one of the main streets in the city. It was one of those typical Canadian winter days, overcast and snowing lightly. The streets were narrower than usual because of the plows clearing the snow. The road was lined with parked cars reducing it to one lane in each direction. He appeared somewhat intimidated as he moved along, but he was surprisingly calm. Actually, looking back I think he may have been traumatized by the conditions. In an instant, the unthinkable happened. Someone sitting in their parked car decided it was time to get out, so he opened the door wide and moved out of the car. It was too late and too slippery to apply the brakes, and I don't think Steven even realized what was happening. Once again I grabbed the steering wheel and swerved towards the oncoming traffic narrowly missing the man but allowing him to drive home that day with all four doors of his vehicle intact.

Steven was sure I was going to yell at him and threaten never to take him on the road again. However, I assured him it wasn't his fault; he had not done anything wrong. The fault of course was the person who hadn't checked the traffic before getting out of his car, recklessly putting himself and others in harm's way. "That's why," I told Steven, "you always need to be prepared for the unexpected and have an escape plan ready, thus the importance of continually checking the rearview mirror, over your shoulder, and oncoming traffic." We were so proud of him the day he finally passed his driving exam. Amazingly, he accomplished passing his driving test on the first try. Linda and I were shocked but also pleasantly surprised. I was pretty proud of myself too. I had faced dangerous conditions, close encounters with many obstacles, and had come out relatively unscathed. Even our car escaped without a scratch.

> Persons with disabilities do have the ability to drive and engage in most of the same activities as others. They should be encouraged to explore the possibility. Using driving as an example, the first step would be to ask a medical doctor if there is any reason learning to drive would be a possibility. In most jurisdictions, persons with disabilities would be required to take a "flexibility test" to determine if they had the physical ability to operate a motor vehicle safely before qualifying for a license to drive. If they pass this test, they should be encouraged to learn to drive. There are driving schools that employ driving instructors that specialize in teaching persons with disabilities to drive.
>
> There are also special accommodations that are available to assist the driver such as hand-controls, like the "spinner" in Steven's case, to assist with turning the steering wheel.
>
> It is critical for the person with disabilities to understand that his or her reaction time will not be as fast as others. For that reason they must always be alert and focused on their driving. This usually means taking extra time to prepare for turns, lane changes, and braking.

INDEPENDENCE NO MATTER WHAT

No matter where Steven was or what he was doing, he did whatever he could to fit in. An avid hockey fan, I would travel now and then to hockey games in other cities with friends. Steven loved traveling with us and was always the first one to the car. Some cities were more than a two-hour drive from home, making it necessary to stop a few times to allow him to get out of the car to stretch. Long drives increased the risk of painful muscle spasms because his legs were generally immobile. The prospect of excruciating pain never seemed to dampen his enthusiasm as he wanted to travel with the guys and experience the fun involved in road trips. Of course, he was also a big Kitchener Ranger fan like his father and like his grandfather was before he passed away.

Attending games away from home presented challenges as we couldn't always depend on there being accessible seating for Steven. I can only imagine what was going through the minds of the spectators in our section when this young man walking with two crutches was about to make his way to his seat several rows below. Going down the steps was easier for him than climbing up, but to the onlooker it must have been terrifying to watch. Using both crutches he would slowly but deliberately lean forward placing one crutch on the next step down. He then carefully transferred his weight onto that crutch while he dragged one foot off the starting step, gingerly setting it on the step below. At this juncture he looked like he was readying himself for a high dive. As soon as he steadied himself he would drag his other foot down and continue the process over and over until he arrived at his destination, apologizing to each row as he slowly made his way past them. Out of the corner of my eye, I could see the look on their face as they held their breath anticipating imminent disaster. I'm sure they thought I was the most negligent, cruel parent in the building. It took a while to get to our seats so you can appreciate how important it was for him to visit the washroom prior to the descent. Yes, it would have been much simpler, and safer, to simply purchase a seat in the handicapped section but Steven would not consent to being segregated from the rest of his party. He never wanted any special concessions to be made for him.

Going up the steps Steven required some assistance; he used my arm for balance and slowly made his way to the main level. Since he did not have a lot of muscle tone in his one leg, moving it took considerable concentration and an enormous effort. Honestly, no matter which direction he was going, whether it was up or down, I was always very nervous, standing close by in the event of any miscue or slip. However, I let Steven determine whether or not he needed help. Rarely did he ask for any kind of assistance as he cherished his independence at almost any cost.

FACING NEW CHALLENGES

After three years of working extremely hard and sacrificing a lot of his personal time with friends, Steven realized his goal of graduating from college. It wasn't easy, and at times we were sure he would quit, but he didn't. The years of positive reinforcement from his family and friends paid off, and with the help of a caring faculty and staff at Conestoga College he overcame every challenge he faced in the academic world. Now he would face one of the biggest challenges of his life—like every other college or university graduate—was that he now had to find a job.

It is never easy for anyone to find a job after graduation; for Steven it was extremely difficult and at times depressing. When he was able to get an interview, he felt companies were making hiring decisions based on his disability and not considering his ability, potential, or at the very least, the fact that he was a college graduate. In many cases the interviewer was patronizing and insincere. Following weeks of searching, he was finally successful securing a career opportunity with an insurance company. He found out quickly that he was being taken advantage of. He had been hired as a sales representative despite the fact that he didn't own a vehicle. Steven never takes on a task without pouring his heart and soul into it. He put in many hours taking taxi cabs to appointments and meetings, spending hundreds of dollars and receiving no income or expenses for his trouble.

Our biggest fear was that he would get depressed and give up. Who could blame him if he did? My suggestion at the time was for him to take advantage of the training and knowledge he was gaining, while quietly looking for another position, one where he could prove himself as a capable employee. He took our advice and continued putting in a full effort at the insurance company while looking for more meaningful employment. During that period he remained cheerful and confident, viewing his dilemma as a "mismatch" rather than blaming his disability. The important thing was that he never complained and continued putting forth his full effort. However at the same time we knew the situation was beginning to weigh heavily on him.

Finally, he found a position he thought was perfect for him at the time. Despite the negative aspects of working in the insurance business, what that job did teach him was that he had a clear talent in working with people. He certainly liked to talk, but he was a good listener too. He was hired as a sales representative at the Gap. He poured his heart and soul into learning the position and the products, eventually getting to the point where people would come into the store specifically to see him and listen to his recommendations. He did a terrific job, and he loved working with the people in the retail environment. He also was quite good with the children who came into the store with their parents.

THE BIG FALL

It was during his tenure at the Gap that Steven met Tanya Petrozi. Steven liked to be around his friends; he could relax and be himself. There was a group of them that seemed to spend a lot of time with each other in restaurants, at parties, or the karaoke bar. Two of Steven's friends, Sarah and Jeff, had a close friend named Allison. Allison's best friend was a young girl named Tanya. The three of them were modern day match-makers telling Steven about this nice young girl who would be perfect for him while doing the same with Tanya. At every opportunity they would suggest to each of them that they should meet. Neither Steven nor Tanya were actively looking for a relationship at the time, so much to the match-making trio's disappointment, they were unable to create a sense of urgency for the two to meet.

Finally, the perfect "natural" situation arose that allowed the group to have Tanya and Steve meet—a birthday party. It was Allison's birthday and the group planned a surprise party for her, meaning they would be inviting friends of Allison, including Tanya. And so Steven's relationship with Tanya began.

In the beginning they would meet at the local karaoke restaurant, but soon they were going to shows, concerts, and volunteer sessions at the Rotary Centre. They were good for each other and enjoyed being together, even if it was just to sit around and talk.

Friends and family joked about the two of them being joined at the hip because they were always together, separated only by work or school. It was a rare occasion when you would see one without the other. If they weren't going to a movie or hanging out together, they would be talking

CLOSING IN ON THE DESTINATION

to each other on the phone. Their relationship grew stronger by the day as they had so many similar interests and were both fiercely independent.

Tanya worked for her parents at a retail store, usually putting in several hours a day. Since they couldn't talk on the phone during working hours, the anticipation of being together later in the day was always what occupied their minds. Steven would take a taxi from home to her work to wait for her if they were going out to dinner. They were inseparable.

While waiting for Tanya to finish work one afternoon in the winter, Steven decided to go to the restaurant across the street and have a soft drink. When it was time to leave, he made his way to the door. It was just that time of day when the sun was low enough in the sky to overwhelm the vision of a person coming from a dark room. He opened the door and went outside, not realizing there was a step down. The shock of missing a step and the icy conditions that day sent him crashing to the ground. Unable to move, he could do nothing more than lay there in a heap with his crutches several feet away.

Steven waited for what seemed like an eternity for someone to come to his aid. The restaurant owner, informed of the mishap, came out to see if Steven was okay. He was in considerable pain and unable to put any weight on his legs. There was no choice but to get him to the hospital. Steven insisted he didn't need an ambulance; as far as he was concerned he would be okay after a rest. The restaurant owner wasn't quite so optimistic and strongly suggested he get medical attention to make sure nothing was broken. Reluctantly, Steven agreed and the owner called a cab for him and made sure he was comfortable until the taxi arrived. It was very difficult for him to get into the cab, and by that time the pain was almost intolerable.

The wait in the emergency room of the hospital was excruciating; Steven couldn't find a position that would ease the pain. Finally a doctor came in to see him and ordered x-rays on his legs and hips. After several hours, and lots of Tylenol, the doctor finally brought Steven the results: there was nothing broken and he could go home and continue taking the painkillers. The doctor said he would be very sore for the next few days but that he would be okay. Steven didn't believe him and questioned the diagnosis. He had been in many situations in the past regarding his legs and hips; he was fairly sure everything wasn't okay. However, at five o'clock in the morning the doctor prevailed, and Steven was sent home.

Linda and I had been at a concert that night and were aware of his fall but unaware of the seriousness until we called him. Steven for some time has been quite self-sufficient and would go to the hospital on his own if he felt it was necessary. Most of the time he wouldn't let us know until after the fact. The fact that he had spent several hours in the emergency ward at the hospital wasn't a surprise as this length of wait had become the norm. But when he told us he was still very uncomfortable, we were quite surprised he was being released. We told him that we would come pick him up. We had a van and it would be more comfortable than a cab.

Rather than inconvenience anyone, and once again displaying his independence, he told us not to worry about how he was going to get home. He suggested calling a cab. This time we insisted on picking him up because we knew what was going on. He was extremely uncomfortable standing. Bending his legs and putting pressure on his hip was so traumatic, he cried out in pain. This was definitely not normal for him; his tolerance was usually very high. We even insisted on consulting with the doctor who, one last time, insisted there was nothing broken and that it was not necessary to keep Steven in the hospital. The doctor said, "He should expect to be uncomfortable for a few days." This would turn out to be a colossal understatement.

I pulled the van up to the emergency room entrance. Steven was waiting in a wheelchair in obvious discomfort. With the assistance of a hospital orderly, we proceeded to lift him into the van. It took nearly fifteen minutes to help him out of the wheelchair and into a seat in the van. He cried out in pain the entire time as he was unable to find any position that offered relief from the pain. On the drive home, every bump in the road was like a knife cutting into his hip.

Getting Steven into the house was an ordeal we will not soon forget. It took close to thirty minutes to assist him out of the van and into our home. He reacted to every movement no matter how slight, crying out in pain. We were certain the neighbors thought we were torturing the poor boy. Linda and I knew he wasn't overreacting, first because he never did, and second because he was soaked from sweat from the stress and effort of it all. The task was made even more difficult by his inability to help at all; the simple act of touching the ground with his foot amplified the pain. Eventually, with a lot of patience, we were able to get him up to his bed.

Over the next few days, we fed him as many painkillers as we safely could, but nothing seemed to work. On the third day, we called the family doctor who told us to get Steven back to the hospital and that he would order more tests. By this time, Steven was somehow able to cope with the pain and discomfort. In his usual independent manner, he called the hospital and requested the ambulance on his own. Steven's room was on the second floor but the paramedics were able to get him on a gurney and transfer him to the ambulance with considerably more ease than we had been able to manage when we brought him home. The trip to the hospital was more comfortable in the ambulance.

When the ambulance arrived at the hospital, it was forced to wait until the emergency room staff could determine what treatment Steven required. The wait in the ambulance lasted more than an hour. They finally determined he would not be admitted. Since he had received the original diagnosis at the other local hospital, the ambulance was directed there—socialized medicine at its best, I guess. Steven was extremely uncomfortable after lying in the ambulance all that time. He was having a lot of difficulty finding a position that offered even a little relief from the pain. With each adjustment in his position, he would cry out. We were unaware of the delays, and when we were informed of the situation, we were furious. We couldn't understand how the hospitals could put him through such an ordeal.

By the time Linda and I arrived at the hospital, a specialist had already seen Steven and had just sent him up for x-rays. Soon after the doctor came out to inform us that Steven had in fact broken his hip and was going to require surgery that night. On top of everything else, this meant he would face at least six weeks in a cast from his waist to his ankles.

As Linda and I observed him during this recovery, we were reminded of just how much of a remarkable inspiration Steven could be. He had every reason to be depressed and to feel sorry for himself, but he didn't. Never once did he even consider that his fall was connected to his disability. It was what it was—an accident. Some tried to convince Steven to take legal action against the restaurant, but it was never a consideration for him. He felt that any attempt to implicate the restaurant would be both unfair and dishonest. He fell, end of story! That attitude spoke volumes of who Steven was and what he was about.

Tanya was with Steven throughout his entire recuperation, missing only those times when she was required to be at work. In retrospect we are sure it was the influence of having her in his life that helped carry him through this particular calamity. His spirits were always high, and he still had time to laugh and make plans for the future. I'm not certain, but I'm quite convinced that sometime during his recovery process, Steven figured out he had his future wife at his bedside.

CHAPTER SEVEN

The End of One Journey— The Beginning of the Next

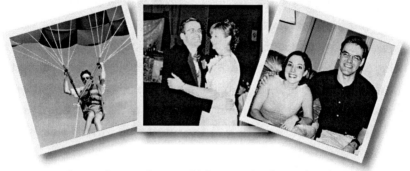

Success is not a place at which one arrives but rather the spirit with which one undertakes and continues the journey.

Alex Noble

In the winter of 1993, on our annual trip to Florida, Steven was with us just as he had been each of the years before. The difference this time was that this trip would be the last one he would take with us as he had finally outgrown the need to be with his parents all the time. The mood of this trip was different from the start; Steven seemed more mature and focused. As we made our way south along the interstate, he rhymed off a litany of new adventures he was going to try. When he was younger, I would have probably acknowledged his claims, responding with a polite, "Really? That would be nice." What I really meant was, "Sure you will!" But this time it was different; this young man knew no fear.

SAILING IN AIR

The list he gave us in the car were adventures I personally would never have tried because of my perceived fear of endangering life and limb. The list included, but was not limited to, bungee jumping, jet skiing, waterskiing, skydiving, and parasailing. He was at the age where I could only offer my sage advice, "Are you crazy? Don't do it!" Linda's advice of course was much more motherly, and practical, and somehow she was able to convince him to narrow his death-defying escapades down to one: parasailing!

I was hoping that by the time we were there for a few days, enjoying the sun and the pool, Steven would forget this death wish. It didn't happen. The minute we arrived at our condo, he was into the brochures and phone book looking for the best parasailing adventure opportunity. I wasn't really embracing this idea and had thoughts of Linda and me being part of a search team scouring the Gulf of Mexico for a youngster who had fallen from the sky. My mind was in panic mode. I envisioned myself trying to describe this brave young soul to the coast guard search and rescue: "Well, officer, he was wearing a blue bathing suit; he has cerebral palsy and walks with crutches."

There were several companies in the Bradenton-Sarasota area that operated parasailing adventures. Steven called each one of them inquiring into the services they offered, the cost, and most importantly, did they have any restrictions? After an hour or so on the telephone, he finally selected the company that was going to launch him hundreds of feet into the air at the end of a tether rope, suspended by a thin sheet of colorful nylon, holding on to a metal bar while being towed by a motor boat. To say he was charged up would be a tremendous understatement. He could hardly sleep waiting for what he was already describing as the most exciting moment of his life.

Two days later, we drove him to the dock on Anna Marie Island where he would meet his parasailing instructor and the team that would take him out into the Gulf. It wasn't until he was actually fitted with his lifejacket that someone on the team asked what seemed to me to be the obvious question: "How are we going to get him into the air, and once the adventure is over, how is he going to land in the water and get picked up in time?" Finally! Someone who had the same concerns as me!

Steven's reply: "Don't worry about it. I can do it!" To my utter amazement, they actually accepted that confirmation without hesitation.

Linda joined Steven on the boat so she could be part of this adventure up close. I couldn't do it and claimed seasickness as an excuse to watch from land. They all believed me and prepared to sail. I headed along the shore in the direction of St. Armand's Circle (Sarasota), where I could have an unobstructed view of this act of insanity. Moments later, there he was. I could see him clearly from my vantage point as he lifted off from the water and climbed high into the air. I was truly amazed. On one hand I was a nervous wreck wishing it was over, on the other, I was overcome with the excitement of watching my son defy the odds. He appeared to be in the air for longer than he contracted for before he started his descent. I began to worry about how they were going to get to him back onto the boat once he landed, but the recovery was routine as they got to him right away, pulling him safely in with only a little difficulty. According to Linda, who of course was bubbling over with pride, he was so excited and pleased with himself. Once again he proved he was capable of doing almost anything he put his mind to and that he was adept at defining his own limitations.

> As parents of children with disabilities we tend to be a little—okay at times very— overprotective. We want to help them avoid every negative experience we can, keep them safe, and shield them from teasing, insensitive comments, and the intolerant attitudes they are certain to experience throughout their lives. This is a natural feeling to have for all our children whether or not the have a disability.
>
> The secret is learning to let go—a little at a time. As difficult as it may seem, the best thing we can do for our children is to let them discover their limitations. If they fail in their attempt to master an activity and experience, they will still profit from the experience and grow stronger. The earlier in life they learn how to deal with setbacks, the stronger they will become as they mature. How they deal with disappointment will strengthen their character and define who they are.

This experience has come to be a defining moment in Steven's life. It was the point where Steven brought together all that we had tried to teach him about living a normal life, and not being afraid to try something new. The end result to him would be—I can do anything! From that moment on, he was a young man who could face uncertainty with courage and conviction and accept the consequences.

I learned a valuable lesson that day as well. I learned that if you truly trust someone, you have to learn to let go and actually let them try. I also learned that Steven truly did know his limitations, far better than I. From that day I have never questioned him when he described an activity that he wanted to participate in. He still asks for advice and we still give it; but we trust he will make the right decisions for himself. He does too.

KARAOKE AND ROMANCE

Back in his college days, Steven developed a strong love for music. He can definitely hold a tune, and he seemed to be able to connect with others through singing. He spent a great deal of time at a local karaoke bar where he found others who shared his enthusiasm for singing. Every Saturday night he would spend endless hours, microphone in hand, singing everything from hard rock to Neil Diamond. On several occasions he participated in elimination contests usually finishing up near the top of the performers. He had found a passion and an activity in which he could compete on a level playing field, without artificial barriers, and he was successful. He made many friends, and reconnected with several old ones from his high school days. He also met Tanya at the karaoke bar along with Jeff Poolton, the same Jeff who helped set them up. Jeff and Steven became best friends and Jeff would be the best man at their wedding.

"Karaoke was very much the focal point of my social life. I met the most important person in my life, my wife, at the Silver Spur, a local restaurant and bar. The Silver Spur was like a home away from home for me. I enjoy karaoke because I've always had an interest in music although I never studied it. I remember I was a bit nervous at first but I knew I could do it; I just needed to gather up my courage. Well, I tried it and did well and I have loved it ever since," Steven shared with me.

THE END OF ONE JOURNEY—THE BEGINNING OF THE NEXT

Once Steven and Tanya met, they appeared to everyone as the perfect couple. It was obviously love at first sight. Tanya recalls, "The first time I saw Steve I liked his smile; he's a good-looking man. When we first met, we talked all night. It didn't take long before I realized we had so much in common. Both of us were very close to our families, we both had a keen interest in helping others, and we both enjoyed traveling. I remember feeling so comfortable around him. I was hoping he would ask me out. Not long after our first meeting, he did call and asked me to dinner. I remember being so excited.

"We were to meet at a restaurant and he was over an hour late. At first I thought he had changed his mind, but I decided to wait for him. It was worth the wait—we spent the evening talking about our friends and families and the things we liked and those we didn't like. I thought I would test him right away, so during our dinner I told him I wanted him to come home with me and meet my parents. Steve was nervous, but at the same time he was still trying to impress me, so he agreed.

"I knew everything was going to be okay as soon as Steven started joking with my father about his hometown of Windsor, [Ontario] across the river from Detroit. Steven found out that both our fathers were staunch Detroit Red Wings fans, so we were off to a great start."

Steven and Tanya both attended the KidsAbility Centre for Child Development as youngsters but they hadn't known each other there because they had attended at different times. They were the first "couple" from the center. Many graduates of the school and therapy programs did marry. It was all very exciting, and Steven finally proposed to Tanya about two years after they met. Steven and Tanya's was the first marriage of two students from within the center's programs.

Jeff helped Steven write a song for Tanya for their wedding, "You Inspire Me." Jeff is a professional singer and Steven worked with him to create his first recording of Tanya's song. Jeff performed the song at their wedding. Jeff and Steven also share a common bond. Both are physically challenged and both have strong positive attitudes. Physical challenges would never hold either one of them back once they focused on an idea or future plan. The two of them always remind me of a golf shirt I wear that proudly states, "Attitude is Everything."

Steven was very influential in Jeff's life as well. "Two words come to mind when thinking about Steve," says Jeff, "generosity and optimism. Steve's never hesitated to give everything he could to someone in need and never seemed to expect anything in return. He always tries to keep me looking at the bright side of every difficult situation. I can remember numerous, serious conversations that somehow ended up in a good laugh. Somehow you just can't stay in a bad mood when Steve's around."

Everyone was thrilled that Steven and Tanya were getting married, and everyone was invited. It was a beautiful day, and I don't think there was a dry eye in the house when Jeff sang Steven's song to his new bride:

"You Inspire Me"

Ever since I met you, I feel so new.
You changed my life and made all my dreams come true.
You're the brightest star in my sky;
I can see heaven when I look into your eyes.
There's nothing like having you by my side.
Whenever you need me I'll be there.
I'll be your biggest fan. I'll do the best I can.
There's no place I'd rather be
    Than by your side.
You inspire me.
And my world's changed because of you
    And there's nothing I wouldn't do.
I've never loved anyone like you.
Look how far we have come.
You know that you're the only one.
Baby, I love you and I will for evermore.
Together I know we'll go so far . . . I hope you always know how
    beautiful you are.
There's nothing like having you in my heart.
There's no place I'd rather be
    Than by your side.
You inspire me

THE END OF ONE JOURNEY—THE BEGINNING OF THE NEXT

And my world's changed because of you
And there's nothing I wouldn't do.
I've never loved anyone like you.

JUST HIMSELF

Steven's aunt, Joan Hackl, who has always been impressed by him and his outlook on life says, "No matter how tough things seem to get for him, he never burdens anyone else with his troubles and never accepts defeat. Ever since Steven was a little boy, two words have never been part of his vocabulary: 'can't do!' Although he looks challenged to others he meets in his daily life (and he is), to himself he is just Steven. He looks into a different mirror than you or I. The face that looks back at him never shows defeat; it is determined and self-confident. Recently he joined a gym, but when I asked him how it was going, he laughed and said something to the effect that it wasn't for him! The one thing he didn't show was a feeling of defeat. To quote my late brother-in-law, 'the thing that stands out most about Steven is, in spite of the hand that was dealt to him, you never hear him complain or say why me? He always has a smile on his face, no matter what.'"

GIVING BACK

We always tried to teach our children that if you give freely of yourself without any expectation of something in return, your life will be enriched and you will profit from it in other ways. Our philosophy was, "The good deeds you do will not go unnoticed."

Volunteering, I am most proud to say, has become a huge part of Steven's life. He could never be accused of not being a generous person. In fact, he is generous to a fault. When he was working part-time, he donated money to every cause that came along. One of the companies he worked for participated in an annual charity fund-raising event permitting employees to pledge donations through payroll deductions. Consistently he gave more than any other part-time employee and at times matched the donations of full-time staff. I'm sure at tax time the government must have wondered if this person was for real.

At times we felt Steven was perhaps too benevolent with his giving spirit. As he grew older, he found a new way to volunteer when he discovered the Canadian Red Cross. While in the hospital for one of his many surgical procedures, he heard the nurses talking about the critical shortage of blood, leaving many patients at risk. Steven's blood type is in high demand with the Red Cross. He proudly displays the collection of pins and letters of commendation he has received in recognition of the number of times he has been a donor. Like every other volunteer experience, he took the shortage of blood very seriously. If he couldn't arrange a ride, he would take a taxi to the clinic and back home. He didn't want it on his conscience if someone needed his blood, and it wasn't available because he didn't make an effort to get to the clinic. On one occasion he was actually turned away as he had donated the maximum amount of blood allowed during the year.

> Most research on cerebral palsy today is focused on traumatic events at birth, and evaluating and developing experimental therapy treatments as well as prevention. The prevention research focuses on blood related issues such as compatibility and prenatal care. However, very little research is being carried out on the effects of cerebral palsy as an individual grows older. There are many questions regarding how aging impacts on the symptoms of persons with the condition? Do the symptoms intensify as the individual gets older? With limited support and resources available for adults with cerebral palsy, the need for research has becomes more critical.

As a young adult, Steven remained strongly committed to giving of himself. He became involved with a community organization that provided support for families who were going through difficult times. They may have been struggling with unemployment, living in poverty, or trying to cope with difficult family situations. Volunteers would assist by spending quality time with one of the children, taking them out to the movies, bowling, or some other activity that would give some relief to the parents and also provide the child with experiences they normally would not have.

THE END OF ONE JOURNEY—THE BEGINNING OF THE NEXT

During his college days, Steven never lost his connection with the KidsAbility Centre, volunteering whenever he could find some time. He never said no if he was asked to participate in a special program or event. He always felt a sense of loyalty to the center, a personal conviction he had to pay back all that the center had done for him in his youth. Many times he went above and beyond the usual expectations of a volunteer, changing his school schedule in order to accommodate a need. He found great personal satisfaction in his volunteering, never expecting to receive any special recognition. His intentions were always selfless and honorable.

Steven Swatridge is the Executive Director of KidsAbility. He has known Steven for several years and witnessed his growth and maturity from his teenage years through to adulthood. "I first met Steven Hendry when he was a teenager about to graduate from KidsAbility, formerly the Rotary Children's Centre. Our paths seldom crossed in those days as he was focused on school and just being a teenager. However, many years later I began seeing Steven on Friday nights at the Kitchener Rangers hockey games. He was often in the company of a young lady named Tanya, whom I had known for over fifteen years. As they appeared together with increasing frequency, it dawned on me that they shared more than a love for hockey. As their relationship matured, I began seeing Steven and Tanya at different KidsAbility events. They were both KidsAbility graduates who had returned as volunteers, eager to contribute back to an organization that they felt had played a significant role in both their lives.

"In his many volunteer roles for KidsAbility, Steven always carried himself as a positive, articulate ambassador for KidsAbility. He assisted with various public events, gave personal testimonials, and acted as a mentor for young people with disabilities. Steven's personal charm, warmth, and passion for life all contributed to his effectiveness as an ambassador for KidsAbility and as a beacon for all people with disabilities and challenges in life. As a result of Steven's many volunteer activities, I've been fortunate to get to know him as a former client, and more importantly, as a young man. I am so impressed with his maturity, confidence, and integrity. He pursues life with passion, exhibits a deep sense of humanity and concern for others, and simply exudes love and support for his wife, Tanya. These are qualities we all want to see in our children, and I expect his parents are deeply proud of the young man he has become.

"Steven's gifts as a volunteer and as a person led to his appointment to the KidsAbility Board of Directors in June of 2008. In that capacity he has contributed his unique perspective and deep concern for people with disabilities and other challenges. He is an effective and articulate spokesperson for the organization, and I look forward to seeing him undertake more challenging leadership roles in the future. I am blessed to call him a colleague and a friend."

As far as Steven is concerned, he feels that serving on the KidsAbility Board of Directors gives him the opportunity to contribute the best way he can—by giving of himself. Steven particularly enjoys working with the teen groups at the center. It never takes him long to get the kids sharing stories and experiences and chatting about their lives. Just having someone to talk to who understands and can relate to what they are feeling is all they need. However, to suggest it is a group of teenagers with disabilities merely sitting around conversing would not be a fair description of their evening. Teenagers are teenagers, no matter their color, religion, cultural difference, or (dis)abilities, so their evenings are also filled with laughter, loud music, some dancing, and lots of snacks.

Tanya, not surprisingly, has also made volunteering a huge part of her life. When she and Steven met, she had been involved for sometime as a sort of "big sister" (as a special friend) with a young girl I'll call Beth. Beth was receiving assistance from a local community support group that provided resources such as "special friends" to families and individuals with special needs. Steven admired the work Tanya was doing with Beth and decided to volunteer with that organization if they would give him the chance. Always the opportunist, he wanted to spend more time with Beth and I'm sure with Tanya as well. He quickly became a source of additional support for Beth.

THE END OF ONE JOURNEY—THE BEGINNING OF THE NEXT

Of the almost four years he spent with that organization, Steven said, "My role was to mentor young people with special needs by helping them develop life skills through a variety of social activities. I decided to join the organization in order to keep working with Beth. The transition from friend to client was easy. The goals that were set for me by my caseworker were to provide respite for Beth's parents, help her develop social skills through activities, and to help her increase the use of one of her limbs. I was working full-time back then and thankfully my schedule allowed me the freedom to spend a few hours a week with her. It was the perfect opportunity for me, and it provided some stability for Beth.

"The Friday-night hockey games seemed to be the perfect social environment where people of all ages and walks of life could gather and enjoy an evening. I thought it might be the perfect environment for Beth to get used to being in large crowds without actually having to communicate with too many of them. Her mother was naturally not as enthusiastic; she was concerned that Beth had struggled with being in crowds in the past, feeling quite uncomfortable. I convinced them both to at least try it one time; if she didn't like it, or became too anxious, we could leave.

"The first game went better than expected; Beth enjoyed watching the game but at the same time was very quiet. As the game progressed, she started asking more and more questions about the rules and the game in general. It was an instant hit with her. Over time she began talking to those around her, asking many of the same questions she had asked me, but it was a major breakthrough for her and a sense of accomplishment and pride for me.

"Eventually Tanya and I would take her to games out of town, and she would spend time chatting with just about anyone that would listen. Beth also needed time to talk about the things that were on her mind about home and school. Giving her a chance to talk to someone outside the home dramatically improved her attitude at home and at school. She had come a long way since we had first met. I knew the time would come when she would want to be spending more time with people her own age or my work would not allow me the time to spend with her like in the past; eventually that time came."

I am grateful for many things, and I am most certainly proud of all that my boys have accomplished in their lives. I must say though, that volunteering is one of the most gratifying of all Steven's accomplishments. Here's someone who could have easily chosen to be a victim, blame everything on his disability, be a burden to all those around him. Steven to his credit never did any of that. Not only that, he has found a way to pass on all that he has learned to other disabled kids, giving them the chance to grow, to find a life outside of the shell of their "special needs." I'm sure he will never stop volunteering, paying forward all he has been given in his life. I am sure he will find riches beyond his imaginings, and he deserves everything he ever gets back in return.

ONE BRAVE SOLDIER

Our family has always been quite close, both in distance and relationships, so it would be fair to say that every family member, to some degree, has influenced Steven and the way in which he approached life. His development over the years, along with his resiliency, left an impression on his cousin, "Aunt" Maureen McNab, Heather's mom. She said, "Steven has been a soldier his whole life. I have never seen anyone quite as brave as Steve and no matter what his problems have been or will continue to be, I personally have only seen a smile on his face. I think the Tin Man would be proud to have Steven's heart and the Lion his bravery. His sense of humor is what has guided him through a life that, at times, was difficult for him. Fortunately, his family has tested his limits in that respect, always giving him unconditional support and encouragement, inspiring him to push himself beyond limits. It is my opinion, that Steven's ability to deal with adversity is due in part to his parents and family. I love this guy a lot and feel very blessed to have had the pleasure of knowing him. I also have to say the many times he has fallen he has given us one heck of a laugh (when he wasn't hurt, of course)!"

Family support is critical in the development of any child. However, family support in the raising of a child with challenges is paramount. A

THE END OF ONE JOURNEY—THE BEGINNING OF THE NEXT

healthy environment including family and friends dramatically increases the potential for success in every child. The desire to stretch beyond perceived abilities becomes a natural phenomenon in every facet of their lives, including their playing, education, and even making plans for the future.

The journey for Steven hasn't ended. In fact, it's just beginning. His life up to this point has been a series of struggles and mountains to climb. He has also enjoyed many victories as he met those challenges head-on and persevered. His attitude and resilience has never ceased to amaze me. There have been many times when I have faced setbacks and difficulties in my life, times that I felt like giving up only to think of Steven and realize my problems were trivial. As I said early on in this book, he has been one of the most positive influences in my life.

Steven accepted his disability many years ago, but in accepting it, he never let it define him. He never appears to give his physical limitations

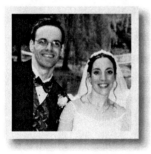

a second thought as he goes about his busy, daily life making plans for the future while dealing with the day-to-day responsibilities of his job and his marriage, demonstrating beyond any doubt that he is uniquely normal.

To the Beginning—Steven & Tanya Hendry

CHAPTER EIGHT

They Defied the Odds so Anything is Possible

I refuse to allow a disability to determine how I live my life. I don't mean to be reckless, but setting a goal that seems a bit daunting actually is very helpful toward recovery.

Christopher Reeve

There can be no doubt that achieving success or rising to the top in any chosen field is never easy. Many challenges must be overcome along the way—acquiring the necessary education, developing the proper skills, seeking opportunity everywhere, and facing competition. In many situations it can also mean rising above the detrimental influence of well-meaning, but negative friends, family members, or employers. These challenges are faced by every person with a dream or a passion to succeed.

For those individuals with disabilities, the mountain to climb is even higher and steeper. They must not only meet the challenges mentioned above, they must also overcome their disability, and in many situations surmount roadblocks such as prejudice, stereotyping, and ignorance. Society has made much advancement in terms of giving all people, disabled or not, the same opportunities, but unfortunately it has a long way to go. There are still companies and people in positions of authority who see the disability first and not the ability, allowing it to influence their decision. Hopefully attitudes will continue to change, allowing more people with physical challenges to reach their full potential.

If you are reading this and you have a disability, or you are the parent of a disabled child, don't despair. I can't stress this enough. In the face of all the negative, don't dismay. A positive, rewarding future is possible with a lot of hard work. Meeting some of these challenges in life head-on will actually create a stronger candidate for success. There are thousands of people with disabilities who have conquered these challenges through hard work, commitment, and unyielding determination, and they have gone on to enjoy very successful careers and lives.

I have often called Steven "uniquely normal," but he really isn't unique in his ability to face and overcome the challenges he has. The following is a list of individuals with various exceptionalities who were unrelenting in overcoming the obstacles in their lives. These individuals never gave up before they achieved success in their chosen field. Each of them has an inspirational story to tell. I give you this list so that you know that success is possible if you believe and persevere. They defied the odds. So can you!

Josh Blue (November 27, 1978) comedian. It is fitting to begin this list with Josh Blue as he epitomizes possibilities by not allowing others to define who he is. Born in the Cameroon with cerebral palsy, Josh is a delightful stand-up comic who immediately engages his audiences with his self-deprecating humor. He is a shining example and inspiration for all persons with disabilities. He has appeared on Comedy Central's *Mind of Mencia, Live with Regis and Kelly, Comics Unleashed,* as well as appearances on Fox, CBS, ABC, and MSNBC. He was the first stand-up comic to appear on *The Ellen DeGeneres Show*. Blue was quoted as saying he wanted "to make people aware of the fact that people with disabilities can make an impact." He is not only an accomplished comedian he is also an athlete participating on the 2004 U.S. Paralympics soccer team. He has tried his hand at painting and even creates sculptures. If that isn't enough, he has also had an acting role, appearing in a low-budget horror film titled *Feast 3: The Happy Finish*. Josh Blue resides in Denver, Colorado.

Rene Kirby (February 27, 1955–), an American film and television actor, appeared in the Farrelly Brothers' film *Shallow Hal,* where he played Walt, a man with spina bifida who led a normal life. Kirby in real life has spina bifida. In high school he was a state champion gymnast. He is also a very capable skier, at times competing in disabled skiing events. He has been known to ski while doing a handstand. One of Rene's quotable quotes—"You don't have to stand up to stand out in a crowd."

Stephen Hawking (January 8, 1942–), professor and world-renowned British theoretical physicist, he is the distinguished research chair at the University of Waterloo's Perimeter Institute for Theoretical Physics (Waterloo, Ontario). Shortly after arriving in Cambridge (England) in 1962, he started developing symptoms of amyotrophic lateral sclerosis (ALS), otherwise known as Lou Gehrig's disease, which would eventually cost him all neuromuscular control. By 1974, he was unable to feed himself, and in 1985 caught pneumonia and had to have a tracheotomy, leaving him unable to speak. Stephen Hawking was the first quadriplegic to float in zero-gravity marking the first time in forty years that he was able to move freely without his wheelchair. Among his many distinctions, Hawking was made a Commander of the Order of the British Empire in 1982.

Franklin Delano Roosevelt (January 30, 1882–April 12, 1945), thirty-second President of the United States, was in power during the Great Depression and World War II and became famous for his "New Deal," which offered relief to the unemployed through recovery of the economy and reform of the banking industry. While vacationing at Campobello Island in New Brunswick, he contracted an illness thought at the time to be polio. He became paralyzed from the waist down. Roosevelt refused to accept the fact that he was paralyzed and only used a wheelchair in private. In public he wore iron braces and walked with a cane. In later years it was determined his illness may not have been polio but Guillain-Barré syndrome.

Steven Fletcher (June 17, 1972–), statesman, is the first quadriplegic to be elected to the Canadian House of Commons, appointed the minister of state in October 2008. He became disabled following a motor-vehicle accident in northern Manitoba when his car hit a moose. Doctors originally told Fletcher he would spend the rest of his life in an institution as he requires round-the-clock attendant care. Later, he would joke about the doctors' comments suggesting he didn't think they meant the institution would be Parliament. Fletcher loves to be in the wilderness, and since his disability, he has worked very hard on recovery and adapting. An inspiration to any individual with a disability, he has competed in water races and won awards using "sip and puff" steering technology. He also has been able to resume his enjoyment of the outdoors through the use of a TrailRider, which allows quadriplegics the ability to travel over rough terrain. Always sporting a positive attitude and sense of humor, of his disability he says, "I would rather be paralyzed from the neck down than the neck up."

Stevie Wonder (May 13, 1950–), singer, songwriter, and musician, has been blind since birth, his condition caused by premature birth (retinopathy of prematurity). Not letting his disability slow him down, Wonder took up the piano at age seven and mastered the instrument by the time he was nine. As if this wasn't enough of a challenge, he learned how to play the harmonica and drums as well. His musical accomplishments during his life are legend. He is also a civil rights activist and the father of seven children.

Andrea Bocelli (September 22, 1958–), Italian tenor, lost his sight at age twelve as a result of glaucoma, a condition he's had since birth. He won his first singing competition at age fourteen. His love of music led him to learn how to play the piano, flute, saxophone, trumpet, harp, trombone, guitar, and drums. Bocelli entered law school after graduating from high school and went on to spend time as a court-appointed lawyer. While too numerous to list, his musical accomplishments include performances for the Pope and former President of the United States, Bill Clinton.

John Mellencamp (October 7, 1951–), singer, songwriter, and musician, was born with a mild form of spina bifida. Mellencamp had a troubled youth, but despite the setbacks he endured, he remained focused and defiant. His music focuses on protest movements, civil liberties, and social awareness. He is also an activist and one of the founders of Farm Aid, a group dedicated to increasing the awareness of the loss of family farms in the US, and raising money through concerts to help families keep their farms. He was inducted into the Rock and Roll Hall of Fame on March 10, 2008.

Samuel L. Jackson (December 21, 1948–), actor. Jackson had a debilitating stutter as a young boy, which he successfully overcame after he took up acting on the advice of his speech therapist. As a young man he was very active in the civil rights movement. All things considered, Jackson's success is quite remarkable considering the setbacks he suffered as a young actor. His career blossomed after his role in *Pulp Fiction*. Other roles include *Rules of Engagement, Changing Lanes, Unbreakable,* and *Shaft*.

Carrie Fisher (October 21, 1956–), actor, screenwriter, and novelist. She is best known for her role as Princess Leia in the original *Star Wars* movie trilogy. Her bestselling novel *Postcards from the Edge* is her most famous literary work and it went on to become a movie in 1990. Fisher has battled a bipolar disorder for several years.

Michael J. Fox (June 9, 1961–), Canadian actor, starred as Alex Keaton in *Family Ties* and Marty McFly in the *Back to the Future* series. He is also known for his voiceovers in such movies as *Stuart Little* and *Homeward Bound: The Incredible Journey*. He is married to actor Tracy Pollan and they have four children. Fox developed symptoms of Parkinson's disease in 1990 and was diagnosed a year later. He has become a strong, outspoken advocate for persons with Parkinson's and founded the Michael J. Fox Foundation, created to research every potential path to finding a cure. Mr. Fox is well known for his support for stem cell research. He has been an outstanding voice and a tremendously positive example of an individual that has overcome the symptoms of his disability in order to fight for change that will help others.

OTHER FAMOUS PEOPLE IN HISTORY, WITH DISABILITIES

Galileo Galilei (February 15, 1564–January 8, 1642) Astronomer, mathematician, philosopher—vision impairment, blindness

John Milton (December 9, 1608–November 8, 1674) Poet—blindness

Sir Isaac Newton (January 4, 1643–March 31, 1727) Astronomer—stuttering

Ludwig van Beethoven (December 17, 1770–March 26, 1827) Composer, conductor, and virtuoso pianist. Suffered gradual hearing loss and became deaf late in his life.

Horatio Nelson (September 29. 1758–October 21, 1805) British admiral—partial blindness

Louis Braille (January 4, 1809–January 6, 1852) Inventor—blindness, the result of stabbing himself accidentally with an awl

Abraham Lincoln (February 12, 1809–April 15, 1865) President of the United States—mood disorder

Harriet Tubman (c. 1820–March 10, 1913) Human rights activist—vision impairment and seizures caused by severe wounds to her head inflicted by a slave owner

Claude Monet (November 14, 1840–December 5, 1926) Impressionist artist—blindness

Thomas Edison (February 11, 1847–October 18, 1931) Inventor—hearing impairment

Winston Churchill (November 30, 1874–January 24, 1965) Prime Minister of England—speech impediment

Jimmy Stewart (May 20, 1908–July 2, 1997) Actor—stuttering

Hank Williams, Senior (September 17, 1923–January 1, 1953) Singer, songwriter—born with an undiagnosed spina bifida occulta

Marilyn Monroe (June 21, 1926–August 5, 1962) Actor—mood disorders, depression

Johnnie Ray (January 10, 1927–February 24, 1990) Singer—hearing impairment

Ray Charles (September 23, 1930–June 10, 2004) Singer, songwriter—blindness

Mel Tillis (August 8, 1932–) Singer, songwriter—stuttering

Brian Wilson (June 20, 1942–) Singer, songwriter—depression

John Denver (December 31, 1943–October 12, 1997) Singer, songwriter—mood disorder

Billy Joel (May 9, 1949–) Singer, songwriter—depression

Bruce Willis (March 19, 1955–) Actor—stuttering

Drew Carey (May 23, 1958–) Comedian—depression

Teddy Pendergrass (March 2, 1950–) Singer, songwriter—paralyzed as a result of a car accident

NOTE: Information, details, dates, and personal details regarding the lives and disabilities of the individuals listed above have been gleaned from a variety of publicly accessible sources including radio and television, newspapers, and the Internet. Their appearance in this chapter is solely for the purpose of providing hope and inspiration to children and adults with disabilities, and their families.

About The Author

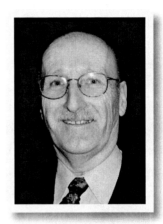

John P. Hendry is not a "technical expert" when it comes to children with special needs. His expertise has been developed over many years of hands-on experience. For more than twenty years he has been an elected school trustee on one of Canada's largest public school boards. Throughout his entire twenty-one years as a trustee he has been a strong, outspoken advocate for all children with challenges serving on the board of the Special Education Advisory Committee (SEAC). His commitment to special education and advocacy role was recognized in Canada by the Province of Ontario with a Cabinet Appointment to the Minister's Advisory Committee on Special Education, a position he held for the maximum six-year term. The Advisory Committee consults the Minister on all matters related to the delivery of programs and services to children with special needs throughout the Province of Ontario. Its membership was all-inclusive and included teachers, principals of both elementary and secondary schools, directors of education (superintendents), members of virtually every special needs association, doctors, aboriginal representatives, trustees, Ministry of Education representatives, and various paraprofessionals.

As a writer, he has a broad spectrum of experience. His accomplishments include a published article in *Hockey Magazine*, a US based publication, The *Hockey News*, *Hockey Journal*, and a two-year term on the community editorial board of a daily newspaper in Kitchener, Ontario. As a member of the Editorial Board he contributed regular columns and editorials. He has also written a paper comparing trends in the

United States and Canadian educational systems, presented at Cal State University in Pasadena, California.

His passion for becoming an advocate for children with challenges was due in part to his youngest son being born premature with cerebral palsy.

Writing a practical, non-technical book for parents of children with disabilities has been a goal of his for many years. Who else but a parent of a child with challenges is in a better position to offer guidance and help to other parents facing the same future? As a professional speaker, he is a member of the Canadian Association of Professional Speakers and the International Federation for Public Speaking. He has addressed groups in Japan, the United States, and Canada. He continues to advocate on behalf of parents of children with disabilities and special education programs and services and most recently was a featured presenter at the Pacific Rim International Conference on Disabilities.

Appendix

Positive Words to Guide You

The greatest you can do for another is not just to share your riches but to reveal to him his own.

Benjamin Disraeli

Here is a list of words that I have found helpful throughout the years raising Steven. It's a list I wanted to share with you so that you, too, can be inspired and motivated to not only succeed in your own life but also help others succeed in theirs.

Accept—Accept advice from others, and consider it in making your decisions and choices. However, never let others make choices for your child.

Believe—Believe that your child will be successful in life, and make all your decisions and plans based on that belief.

Faith—Have faith that your child will be ready to be independent by the time she becomes a young adult.

Confidence—Build your child's confidence at every stage of their life. Monitor his participation at school to insure that his programs are helping to build confidence. Whenever possible, encourage him to become involved in extra-curricular programs.

Perseverance—Never stop pushing to insure your child receives every possible opportunity to participate in mainstream activities (if that is possible within her ability). Remember, there are still many people out there who feel they are doing the right thing by not asking your child to participate. Make the phrase "You can do it!" your mantra. Encourage your child every day to stretch beyond her present abilities.

Dream—Seize every opportunity to dream big dreams, and motivate your child to do the same. Reach for the sky! Dreams can come true, but not without your help and a lot of determination.

Trust—Trust in those who are truly interested in your child's future. Consider their advice. If you have a professional who does not exude trust, find one that does.

Encourage—Encourage your child to try achieving to the fullest extent of his ability. It is vital your child knows you are behind him all the way. A few words of encouragement every day will eventually create the attitude that he can be successful.

Advocate—Advocate on behalf of your child to insure that she receives the same opportunities as every other child. If your daughter is old enough to know her limitations, let her decide how far she should push herself. If she doesn't know her limitations, you can help her figure it out. Don't let a relative stranger decide what your child is capable of accomplishing. Never let anyone define who your child is or what she capable of accomplishing. The right to make that decision is exclusively hers.

Teamwork—Your child's future can be much brighter if everyone involved in her life is working together as a positive, cohesive team. This means doctors, therapists, family members, friends, and relatives must consistently work toward the same goal, and believe it is possible. A consistent message from her team will create a positive environment for her and eliminate the potential for confusion and self-doubt.

Educate—Educate others, including your child's classmates, friends, and relatives about his challenges. Some progressive teachers encourage special-needs students to do a presentation to the class to help them understand and become more tolerant and accepting. Make an effort to attend parent-teacher meetings. You can learn a lot about the education

APPENDIX: POSITIVE WORDS TO GUIDE YOU

and opportunities your child is receiving. Listen for words or phrases that may suggest school staff do not fully understand your child's exceptionality, or that he is not being included in all class activities.

Hope—No matter how gloomy your child's present situation may appear from time to time, never lose hope that things will change for the better soon. If you believe, there is always hope.

Support—Never feel sorry for yourself when you think of your child, and never ask, "Why me?" It is your child that has challenges—not you! What she needs more than anything else is your love and support. Endeavor to treat your child in exactly the same way you would treat any child, making exceptions only when absolutely necessary.

Passion—Make your child's life your passion. Be ever vigilant that he receives every reasonable opportunity to participate in mainstream activities, and that those activities, or school programs, are accessible for him.

Positive Attitude—It is critical that the child and family have a positive attitude. Facing the challenges ahead at times may seem to be overwhelming. A positive attitude will make the difference in meeting those challenges head on. Having a positive attitude will also help you find ways to cope and develop create solutions.

Inspiration—At every opportunity inspire your child to believe she can stretch and do better, that it's up to her. Never allow anyone to have your child accept less than she is capable of achieving.

Determination—Help your child develop that unstoppable attitude to rise above his limitations and believe that there isn't anything that can stop him from reaching his goal.

Bravery—There will be times in your child's life when being brave may mean that you are the only one who knows that you are afraid. Sometimes you may have to be brave for your child.

Courage—Help your child understand from a very young age the importance of confronting difficulties with courage and a firmness of spirit. This isn't an assurance that everything will turn out the way it was hoped, but the experience will strengthen her character.

Resources, Addresses, and Contacts

The following is a listing of Web sites and e-mail addresses of various organizations that can help disabled and impaired individuals. I provide it for your reference only. Both Canadian and American contacts are listed if available. I have also listed the national sites of associations and other organizations wherever possible. From there you should be able to find links to the state or provincial branches.

In addition you will find a selection of parent support groups and some government programs.

I encourage you to contact the organizations that can help provide you with support and guidance specific to your child's needs. These organizations are here to help; you don't have to navigate this journey on your own.

This list is accurate to the best of my ability as of the date of publication.

American Council of the Blind

Web site: www.acb.org
E-mail: ncrabb@erols.com
American Diabetes Association
Web site: www.diabetes.org

Americans with Disabilities Act of 1990

Web site: www.ada.gov

American Foundation for the Blind (AFB)

Web site: www.afb.org
E-mail: afbinfo@afb.net

American Society for Deaf Children
    Web site: www.deafchildren.org
    E-mail: ASDC1@aol.com

American Speech-Language-Hearing Association (ASHA)
    Web site: www.asha.org
    E-mail: actioncenter@asha.org

Asperger Syndrome Education Network (ASPEN)
    Web site: www.aspennj.org
    E-mail: info@aspennj.org

Asthma and Allergy Foundation of America
    Web site: www.aafa.org
    E-mail: info@aafa.org

Asthma Society of Canada
    Web site: www.asthma.ca
    E-mail: info@asthma.ca

Autism Society Canada
    Web site: www.autismsocietycanada.ca
    E-mail: info@autismsocietycanada.ca

Autism Society of America
    Web site: www.autism-society.org

Brain Injury Association of America
    Web site: www.biausa.org
    E-mail: info@biausa.org

Brain Injury Association of Canada
    Web site: http://biac-aclc.ca
    E-mail: info@biac-aclc.ca

Canadian Association for Community Living
    Web site: www.cacl.ca
    E-mail: inform@cacl.ca

RESOURCES, ADDRESSES, AND CONTACTS

Canadian Association of the Deaf
　　Web site: www.cad.ca
　　E-mail: info@cad.ca

Canadian Diabetes Association
　　Web site: www.diabetes.ca
　　E-mail: info@diabetes.ca

Canadian Down Syndrome Society
　　Web site: www.cdss.ca
　　E-mail: info@cdss.ca

Canadian Education Association
　　Web site: www.cea-ace.ca
　　E-mail: info@cea-ace.ca

Canadian Exceptional Children Association
　　Dissolved December 2008 (See Canadian Education Association)

Canadian Human Rights Commission
　　Web site: www.chrc-ccdp.ca/disabilities

Canadian Lung Association
　　Web site: www.lung.ca
　　E-mail: info@lung.ca

Canadian Mental Health Association
　　(notable for their insistence on not using drug therapy to treat mental illness)
　　Web site: www.cmha.ca
　　E-mail: info@cmha.ca

Canadian National Institute for the Blind
　　Web site: www.cnib.ca
　　E-mail: info@cnib.ca

Canadian Paraplegic Association
　　Web site: www.canparaplegic.org
　　E-mail: info@canparaplegic.org

Canadian Stuttering Association
    Web site: www.stutter.ca
    E-mail: csa-info@stutter.ca

Cerebral Palsy International Research Foundation
    Web site: www.cpirf.org
    E-mail: nmaher@cpirf.org

Childhood Apraxia of Speech Association
    Web site: www.apraxia-kids.org
    E-mail: helpdesk@apraxia-kids.org

Children's Hemiplegia and Stroke Association
    Web site: www.chasa.org
    E-mail: info437@chasa.org

Children's Tumor Foundation
    Web site: www.ctf.org
    E-mail: info@ctf.org

Cornucopia of Disability Information (CODI)
    Web site: http://codi.buffalo.edu

Council for Exceptional Children (CEC)
    Web site: www.cec.sped.org
    E-mail: cec@cec.sped.org

Developmental Delay Resources (DDR)
    Web site: www.devdelay.org
    E-mail: devdelay@mindspring.com

Disability.gov
    Web site: www.disability.gov
    E-mail: webmaster@disability.gov

Easter Seals—Canada
    Web site: http://easterseals.ca
    E-mail: info@easterseals.ca

Easter Seals Ontario
Web site: www.easterseals.org
E-mail: info@easterseals.org

Easter Seals—US
Web site: www.easterseals.com
E-mail: info@easterseals.com

Epilepsy Canada
Web site: http://epilepsy.ca
E-mail: epilepsy@epilepsy.ca

Epilepsy Foundation—National Office
Web site: www.epilepsyfoundation.org

Families for Early Autism Treatment (FEAT)
Web site: www.feat.org
E-mail: webmaster@feat.org

Family Village
Web Site: www.familyvillage.wisc.edu
E-mail: familyvillage@waisman.wisc.edu

Hydrocephalus Association
Web site: www.hydroassoc.org
E-mail: hydroassoc@aol.com

Independent Living Institute (ILI)
Web site: www.independentliving.org
E-mail: admin@independentliving.org

Institute for Community Inclusion (ICI)
Web site: www.communityinclusion.org
E-mail: ici@umb.edu

International Dyslexia Association
Web site: www.interdys.org
E-mail: info@interdys.org

International Resource Center for Down Syndrome
E-mail: hf854@cleveland.freenet.edu

International Rett Syndrome Association (IREA)
Web site: www.rettsyndrome.org
E-mail: irsa@rettsyndrome.org

KidsAbility Centre for Child Development
Web site: www.kidsability.ca

Learning Disabilities Association of America (LDA)
Web site: www.ldanatl.org
E-mail: vldanatl@usaor.ne

Learning Disabilities Association of Canada (LDAC)
Web site: www.ldac-taac.ca
E-mail: info@ldac-taac.ca

March of Dimes Foundation—Ontario (& Canada)
Web site: www.marchofdimes.ca
E-mail: info@dimes.on.ca

March of Dimes Foundation—US
Web site: www.marchofdimes.com
E-mail: askus@marchofdimes.com

Mobility International USA
Web site: www.miusa.org

Multiple Sclerosis Society of Canada
Web site: www.mssociety.ca
E-mail: info@mssociety.ca

Muscular Dystrophy Association (MDA)
Web site: www.mda.org
E-mail: mda@mdausa.org

Muscular Dystrophy Canada
Web site: www.muscle.ca
E-mail: info@muscle.ca

National Association of the Deaf (NAD)
Website: www.nad.org
E-mail: nadinfo@nad.org

National Ataxia Foundation
Web site: www.ataxia.org
E-mail: naf@mr.net

National Center to Improve Practice in Special Education (NCIP)
Web site: http://www2.edc.org
E-mail: judyz@edc.org

National Council on Independent Living (NCIL)
Web site: www.ncil.org
E-mail: ncil@ncil.org

National Disability Rights Network (NDRN)
Web site: www.ndrn.org

National Dissemination Center for Children with Disabilities
Web site: www.nichcy.org
E-mail: nichcy@aed.org

National Down Syndrome Congress (NDSC)
Web site: www.ndsccenter.org
E-mail: info@ndsccenter.org

National Down Syndrome Society (NDSS)
Web site: www.ndss.org
E-mail: info@ndss.org

National Family Association for Deaf-Blind (NFADB)
Web site: www.nfadb.org
E-mail: nfadb@aol.com

National Federation for the Blind
Web site: www.nfb.org
E-mail: nfb@iam.digex.net

National Middle School Association (NMSA)
Web site: www.nmsa.org

National Multiple Sclerosis Society
Web site: www.nationalmssociety.org

National Organization on Fetal Alcohol Syndrome (NOFAS)
Web site: www.nofas.org

National Parent Network on Disabilities (NPND)
E-mail: npnd@cs.com

National Reye's Syndrome Foundation
Web site: www.reyessyndrome.org
E-mail: nrsf@reyessyndrome.org

National School Boards Association
Web site: www.nsba.org

National Scoliosis Foundation
Web site: www.scoliosis.org
E-mail: nsf@scoliosis.org

National Spinal Cord Injury Association
Web site: www.spinalcord.org
E-mail: nscia2@aol.com

National Stuttering Association (NSA)
Web site: www.nsastutter.org
E-mail: nsastutter@aol.com

Ontario Federation for Cerebral Palsy (OFCP)
Note: Worldwide links available through this site
Web site: www.ofcp.on.ca
E-mail: info@ofcp.on.ca

Ontario Rett Syndrome Association
Web site: www.rett.ca

RESOURCES, ADDRESSES, AND CONTACTS

Parents for Children's Mental Health
Web site: www.pcmh.ca
E-mail: admin@pcmh.ca

Parents Helping Parents (PHP) (a parent directed family resource center for children with special needs)
Web site: www.php.com
E-mail: info@php.com

Pathways Awareness Foundation (for children with movement difficulties)
Web site: www.pathwaysawareness.org
E-mail: friends@pathwaysawareness.org

Pedal with Pete (for research on cerebral palsy)
Web site: www.pedalwithpete.com
E-mail: petezeid@aol.com

Recording for the Blind & Dyslexic
Web site: www.rfbd.org
E-mail: custserv@rfbd.org

Special Olympics Canada
Web site: www.specialolympics.ca
E-mail: info@specialolympics.ca

Special Olympics International
Web site: www.specialolympics.org
E-mail: specialolympics@msn.com

Spina Bifida and Hydrocephalus Association of Canada
Web site: www.sbhac.ca
E-mail: info@sbhac.ca

Spina Bifida Association of America
Web site: www.sbaa.org
E-mail: sbaa@sbaa.org

Stuttering Foundation of America
   Web site: www.stutteringhelp.org
   E-mail: info@stutteringhelp.org

Tourette Syndrome Association (TSA)
   Web site: http://tsa-usa.org
   E-mail: ts@tsa-usa.org

Tourette Syndrome Foundation of Canada
   Web site: www.tourette.ca
   E-mail: tsfc@tourette.ca

United Cerebral Palsy (UCP)
   Web site: www.ucp.org
   E-mail: info@ucp.org

World Association of Persons with Disabilities
   Note: Worldwide links available through this site
   Web site: www.wapd,org
   E-mail: wapdchapters@wapd.org

Terms of Disabilities

Oftentimes, when parents take their child to a doctor, the doctor starts listing conditions and such that the parents don't understand. Confusion is the clear result. To offer help in this area, I've included this glossary. The conditions, descriptions, and causes of the terms listed below are not to be considered complete. They are listed to give the reader an overview only. For a complete explanation, the reader should either consult the appropriate organization or a doctor.

Amyotrophic Lateral Sclerosis (ALS): A rare fatal progressive disease caused by the degeneration of motor neurons. The condition is often referred to as Lou Gehrig's Disease in reference to the famous New York Yankees player, Lou Gehrig, who was diagnosed with the condition in 1939 and died from it two years later.

Aphasia: A speech disorder in which there is a loss of ability to express and/or comprehend through verbal and written communication, usually resulting from a stroke or brain damage.

Apraxia: A neurological disorder characterized by loss of the ability to execute or carry out learned purposeful movements despite having the desire and physical ability to perform them. It is a disorder of motor planning that may be acquired or developmental, but is not caused by in-coordination, sensory loss, or failure to comprehend simple commands. Apraxia should not be confused with aphasia, an inability to produce and/or comprehend language, or abulia, the lack of desire to carry out an action. The root word of apraxia is praxis, Greek for an act, work, or deed.

Asperger Syndrome: An autism spectrum disorder. Individuals with Asperger's syndrome usually have difficulty with social interaction, and often demonstrate restricted and repetitive patterns of behavior and interests. Asperger syndrome differs from other forms of autism spectrum disorders in that people with it do not suffer from a lack of linguistic and cognitive development. The exact cause is unknown, although research supports the likelihood of a genetic basis. Brain imaging techniques have not identified an apparent common cause.

Assistive Technology Devices: A generic term that includes assistive, adaptive, and rehabilitative devices for people with disabilities to improve their capabilities.

Ataxia: A neurological sign and symptom resulting in a lack of coordination of muscle movements. Ataxia is a non-specific clinical condition implying dysfunction of parts of the nervous system that coordinate movement.

Ataxic Cerebral Palsy: The least common type of cerebral palsy. Persons with ataxic cerebral palsy have difficulty with balance and depth perception. They usually have poor muscle tone, a staggering walk, and unsteady hands.

Athetoid Cerebral Palsy: Also referred to as "athetosis," this leads to difficulty controlling and coordinating movement. Persons with athetoid cerebral palsy experience many involuntary movements and are constantly in motion. They also can have difficulties with speech.

Atrophy: A partial or complete wasting away of parts of the body. In the case of individuals with cerebral palsy, atrophy sometimes occurs after surgery when muscle tissue is cut or removed, resulting in a weakened condition for the remaining muscle.

Audiology: A service that includes identification, determination of hearing loss, and referral for habilitation of hearing.

Autism: A neurological development disorder characterized by impaired social interaction and communication, and by restrictive and repetitive behavior. These signs usually appear before the child is three years of age.

Behavior Intervention Plan: A plan of positive behavioral interventions in the IEP (Individual Education Plan) of a child whose behavior interferes with his/her learning or that of others.

Cerebral Palsy (CP): Is an umbrella term encompassing a group of non-progressive, non-contagious conditions that cause physical disability in human development. CP is caused by damage to the motor control center of the developing brain and can occur during pregnancy (approximately 75 percent of cases), and during childbirth (approximately 5 percent), or after birth (approximately 15 percent) up to age three. Being a non-progressive disorder, the brain damage does not worsen, but secondary orthopedic difficulties are common.

Deafness: A hearing loss that is a full or partial decrease in the ability to understand sounds. Hearing loss, or deafness, can be caused by a wide range of biological or environmental factors.

Diabetes: A disease in which the body does not produce or properly use insulin. Insulin is a hormone that is needed to convert sugar, starches, and other food into the energy needed for daily functioning.

Type 1 diabetes results from the failure of the pancreas to produce insulin, the hormone that unlocks the cells of the body, allowing the glucose to enter and fuel them. Usually diagnosed in children and adolescents, 10 percent of people with diabetes have this Type 1.

Type 2 diabetes results from insulin resistance (a condition in which the body fails to properly use insulin), combined with regular insulin deficiency. This diabetes develops usually in adulthood.

Gestational diabetes can develop during pregnancy, occurring in about 3.7 percent of all pregnancies. It's a temporary condition but may increase the chances of mother and child developing diabetes.

Pre-diabetes occurs when a person's blood glucose levels are higher than normal but not high enough for a diagnosis of Type 2 diabetes.

Diplegia: A type of cerebral palsy where all four limbs are involved. It differs from quadriplegia in that the legs are more affected than the arms.

Disability: An impairment that substantially affects one or more major life activities.

Down Syndrome: A chromosomal disorder caused by the presence of all or a part of an extra twenty-first chromosome. It is named after John Langdon Down, the British doctor who detailed the disorder in 1866.

Dyslexia: A learning disability that causes difficulty with written language. Someone with this disability would have a particular problem with reading and spelling. It is separate and distinct from reading difficulties caused by other conditions.

Early Intervention: Usually refers to educational services provided to children with exceptionalities under the age of five. The earlier a child's challenges are identified and addressed through intervention the higher the possibility of significant improvement.

Special Education Consultant: An individual with teaching experience who is familiar with curriculum and requirements at various grade levels. Special education consultants would have specific training and educational background in special education programs and services. They may or may not have specific expertise in one or more exceptionalities.

Epilepsy: One of the more common chronic neurological disorders, characterized by recurrent unprovoked seizures. The seizures in epilepsy may be related to a brain injury or family tendency, but often the cause is unknown. The word "epilepsy" does not indicate anything about the cause or severity of the person's seizure.

Exceptional Children: A term used primarily by educators to describe children that have been identified as having one or more exceptionalities. An example might be a child that has a learning disability as well as a physical disability. Usually, additional resources are required in order provide equity in their educational opportunities.

Hemiplegia: A type of cerebral palsy where one side of the body is affected.

Hydrocephalus: A term to describe the abnormal accumulation of cerebrospinal fluid in the ventricles or cavities of the brain. This may cause increased intracranial pressure inside the skull and progressive enlargement of the head, convulsion, and mental disability. Usually hydrocephalus does not cause intellectual disability if recognized and properly treated.

Individual Education Plan (IEP): A document that is prepared by the special education team that identifies the programs and services that will be employed in order to help meet a child's educational needs.

KidsAbility Centre for Child Development: An accredited charitable organization that was formed to help children with disabilities. The facility works with eighteen other similar centers in Ontario. Some of the services provided include, but are not limited to, augmentative communication, autism intervention services, early childhood education, medical services, occupational therapy, physiotherapy, resource center, seating and mobility, social work, speech-language therapy, and therapeutic recreation.

Mainstreaming: When a student with special needs is placed into a regular class. Placements can be for the entire school day or at least part of the school day.

Monoplegia: A type of cerebral palsy where only one limb is affected, usually the arm.

Multiple Disabilities: When a child has two or more exceptionalities; for example, intellectual challenges, orthopedic disabilities, and speech-language deficits that cannot be accommodated in special-education programs that address only one of the impairments.

Multiple Sclerosis (MS): A disabling autoimmune condition in which the immune system attacks the central nervous system, leading to demyelination. MS affects the ability of nerve cells in the brain and spinal cord to communicate with each other. There is no known cure for

MS. Treatments attempt to return function after an attack, prevent new attacks, and slow down progression of the disability.

Muscular Dystrophy (MD): Refers to a group of genetic, hereditary muscle diseases that cause progressive muscle weakness. Muscular dystrophies are characterized by progressive skeletal muscle weakness, defects in muscle proteins, and the death of muscle cells and tissue.

Neurofibromatosis: A genetically inherited condition in which nerve tissue grows tumors that may be harmless or cause serious damage by compressing nerves and other tissues. The disorder affects all neural crest cells. The tumors may cause bumps under the skin, colored spots, skeletal problems, pressure on spinal nerve roots, and other neurological problems.

Occupational Therapy: Therapy that remediates fine motor skills.

Obsessive-Compulsive Disorder Spectrum (OCD): Comprises a hypothesized spectrum of psychiatric and medical disorders thought to be related to obsessive-compulsive disorder. Many of these disorders overlap with OCD in symptomatic profile, demographics, family history, neurobiology, comorbidity, clinical course, and response to various pharmacotherapies. Some proposed OCD spectrum disorders include eating disorders such as anorexia nervosa, bulimia nervosa, autism, Asperger syndrome, and Tourette syndrome, to name a few.

Paraplegia: Paralysis of the lower part of the body including the legs.

Quadriplegia: Paralysis distinguished by the loss of motion, reflexes, and sensation in the trunk of the body, in addition to both legs and arms.

Rett Syndrome: A unique developmental disorder that is first recognized in infancy and is seen most frequently in girls. Rett syndrome causes problems in brain function that are responsible for cognitive, sensory, emotional, motor, and autonomic function. These can include learning, speech, sensory sensations, mood, movement, breathing, cardiac function, and even chewing, swallowing, and digestion.

Reye's Syndrome: Is a potentially fatal disease that causes numerous detrimental effects to many organs, especially the brain and liver. It has been associated with aspirin consumption by children with viral diseases such as chickenpox.

Scoliosis: Believed to be a congenital condition in which a person's spine is abnormally curved from side to side, or rotated. Approximately 4 percent of children between the ages of ten and fourteen have detectable scoliosis, and of that number sixty to eighty percent are girls. Boys are usually affected earlier in childhood.

Spasticity: A condition in which the muscles are rigid, the posture may be abnormal, and fine motor control is impaired. It frequently occurs in people with cerebral palsy.

Speech-Language Impairment: Includes communication disorders, language impairments, and/or voice impairments that adversely affect educational performance.

Speech-Language Pathology Services: A service that includes identification and diagnosis of speech or language impairments, speech or language therapy, counseling, and guidance.

Spina Bifida: A developmental birth defect involving the neural tube. Incomplete closure of the embryonic neural tube results in an incompletely formed spinal cord. In addition, the vertebrae overlying the open portion of the spinal cord do not fully form and remain un-fused and open, causing the abnormal portion of the spinal cord to stick out through the opening in the bones.

Stuttering: A form of dysfluency, it is an interruption in the flow of speech. In most cases stuttering disappears on its own by age five, but in others it lasts longer. There is no cure for the condition but effective treatments are available to overcome it. People who stutter process language in a different part of the brain. Approximately 60 percent of those that stutter are caused by genetics.

Tourette Syndrome: An inherited disorder with onset in childhood, characterized by the presence of multiple physical (motor) tics and at least one vocal (phonic) tic. Tourette syndrome is defined as part of a spectrum of tic disorders, which includes transient and chronic tics. Between one and ten children per one thousand have Tourette's, and as many as ten per one thousand people may have tic disorders with the more common tics of eye blinking, coughing, throat clearing, sniffing, and facial movements.

Triplegia: A type of cerebral palsy where three limbs are involved, usually both arms and a leg.

LaVergne, TN USA
18 May 2010
183020LV00004B/12/P